Tai Chi Chuan

SANKOFA

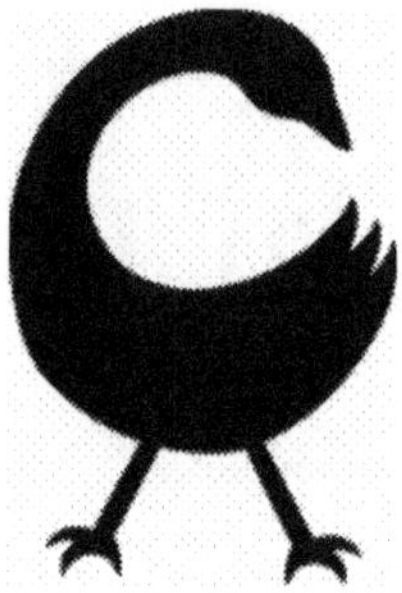

"Se wo were fi na wo sankofa a yenkyi."
(It is not a taboo to go back and retrieve it if you forget.)

Above is one version of the *Sankofa* Adinkra symbol of the Akan people of West Africa. It depicts one bird looking back while walking forward. Others versions may represent two birds facing in opposite directions, or double hearts. *Sankofa* symbolizes retrieving wisdom from the past to take into the future.

Books in the Serikali Sankofa Series

Tai Chi Chuan: An Afriasian Resource for Health and Longevity *(2006)*

Hairlocking: A Guide for the Amateur Locktician (2000)

Tai Chi Chuan

An Afriasian Resource for Health and Longevity

Mfundishi Obuabasa Serikali

iUniverse, Inc.
New York Lincoln Shanghai

Tai Chi Chuan
An Afriasian Resource for Health and Longevity

iUniverse books may be ordered through booksellers or by contacting:

iUniverse
2021 Pine Lake Road, Suite 100
Lincoln, NE 68512
www.iuniverse.com
1-800-Authors (1-800-288-4677)

ISBN-13: 978-0-595-39857-7 (pbk)
ISBN-13: 978-0-595-84255-1 (ebk)
ISBN-10: 0-595-39857-X (pbk)
ISBN-10: 0-595-84255-0 (ebk)

Printed in the United States of America

DISCLAIMER

The author of this book does not dispense medical advice nor prescribe the use of any technique as a form of treatment for medical problems without the advice of a physician, either directly or indirectly. The intent of the author is only to offer information of a general nature to help you cooperate with your doctor in your mutual quest for good health. In the event you use any of the information in this book for yourself, you are using your constitutional right to prescribe for yourself but the author and publisher assume no responsibility for your actions.

Please note that the author and publisher of this book are NOT RESPONSIBLE in any manner whatsoever for any injury that may result from practicing the techniques and/or following the instructions given within. Since the physical activities described herein may be too strenuous in nature for some readers to engage in safely as beginners, it is essential that you consult a physician prior to any training.

All material provided herein is for educational purposes only. Consult your own physician or medical provider to see if the exercises and advice given are appropriate for you. Consult with your qualified medical practitioner regarding the applicability of any opinions or recommendations with respect to your symptoms or medical conditions or diet. Some of the information presented does not necessarily agree with other opinions.

The Food and Drug Administration has not evaluated this information and it is here for you to use at your own discretion.

To

The Proud Few

Who Sacrificed So Much

For So Many

Contents

Foreword xi

Preface xv

Acknowledgements xxi

1 Tai Chi and Mfundishi Obuabasa Serikali 1

2 Tai Chi Traditional History 9

3 Tai Chi Familial Styles 13

4 Tai Chi and the African-Asian Connection 19

5 Tai Chi and Health 27

Photo Gallery* *46

6 Tai Chi & Spirituality 52

7 Tai Chi Technique 66

8 Tai Chi and the Seven Golden Movements 74

9 Tai Chi and Diet 89

10 Tai Chi FAQs 98

Bibliography 109

About the Author 113

Foreword

It is with great pleasure that we offer this short opening to Mfundishi "Baba" Serikali's book, *Tai Chi Chuan: An Afriasian Resource for Health and Longevity.* As novices in the art of practicing Tai Chi, we have come to know, even in this short time, how valuable this can be to our health and general well being.

We have traveled to China, where parks, building roof tops and other gathering spaces host groups—large and small—of people, both young and old, moving in the slow rhythmic movements of Tai Chi. There, watching those many people moving so effortlessly and in unison, we came to realize how beautiful and how thrilling it was to be a part of this global revolution in health maintenance. At the ethereal Temple of Heaven that served the ancient Ming and Qing Dynasties from the early 1400s, there, too, was a large group of people stretching well up into their senior years, moving together in a kind of group meditation. The practice of Tai Chi outdoors is a particularly important aspect of Chinese health and life and here was a group, in the beautiful garden of the Temple of Heaven, tying the natural with the spiritual in mass harmony. Farther along in the park, there was another practitioner, this time a middle-aged woman. A solitary figure with a large sword, she followed some internal beat as she moved sinuously through the form.

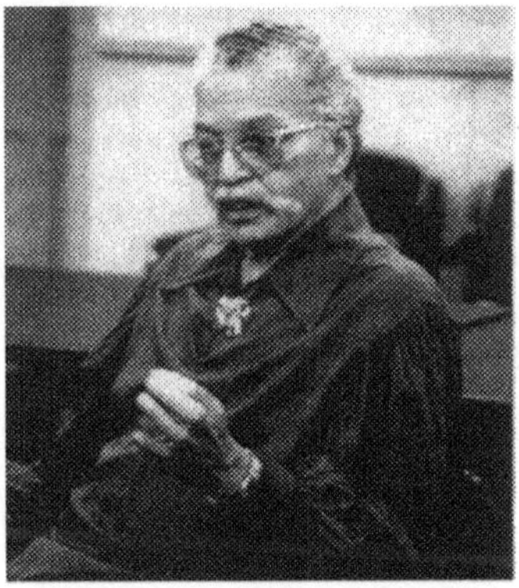

Professor Jan Carew, author of **Ghosts in our Blood**
Photo courtesy of Jan Carew

Mfundishi "Baba" Serikali writes about the origins of Tai Chi in China and its evolutions through time as it has come down to us as his students. He notes its martial arts base, but places a particular emphasis on its health benefits, and indeed people will approach the learning of and practicing of Tai Chi from their own personal need. For me, Jan Carew, it has been a question of finding better ways to manage aging and the growing stiffness of the Parkinson's disease with which I have been afflicted. For me, Joy Carew, it has been a question of finding an oasis from the stressful demands of daily life. Indeed, the time we are practicing Tai Chi, we have—even at this early point—found respite, relief, and rejuvenation.

Indeed, we people of African descent have had longstanding historical and cultural links with China. Returning to the subject of our recent visit to China, we could not help but remember how the famed Dr. W. E. B. DuBois, on his 91st birthday, had in the early 1960s delivered a public address at Peking (now Beijing) University, which was broadcast to thousands upon thousands of people on the African continent. It was there that he had called upon Africa and peoples of African descent to look upon China and its people as their brethren, calling the Chinese "flesh of your flesh and blood of your blood." DuBois knew, like we, that a unity with China would net much learning and that through this unity we would find the strength to build a new day.

We hope that this book will be the beginning for many to consider the health benefits of Tai Chi in this fast-paced world.

Prof. Jan R. Carew,
Emeritus Professor of African American and Third World Studies
Northwestern University

Joy G. Carew, Ph.D.
Associate Professor of Pan-African Studies
University of Louisville

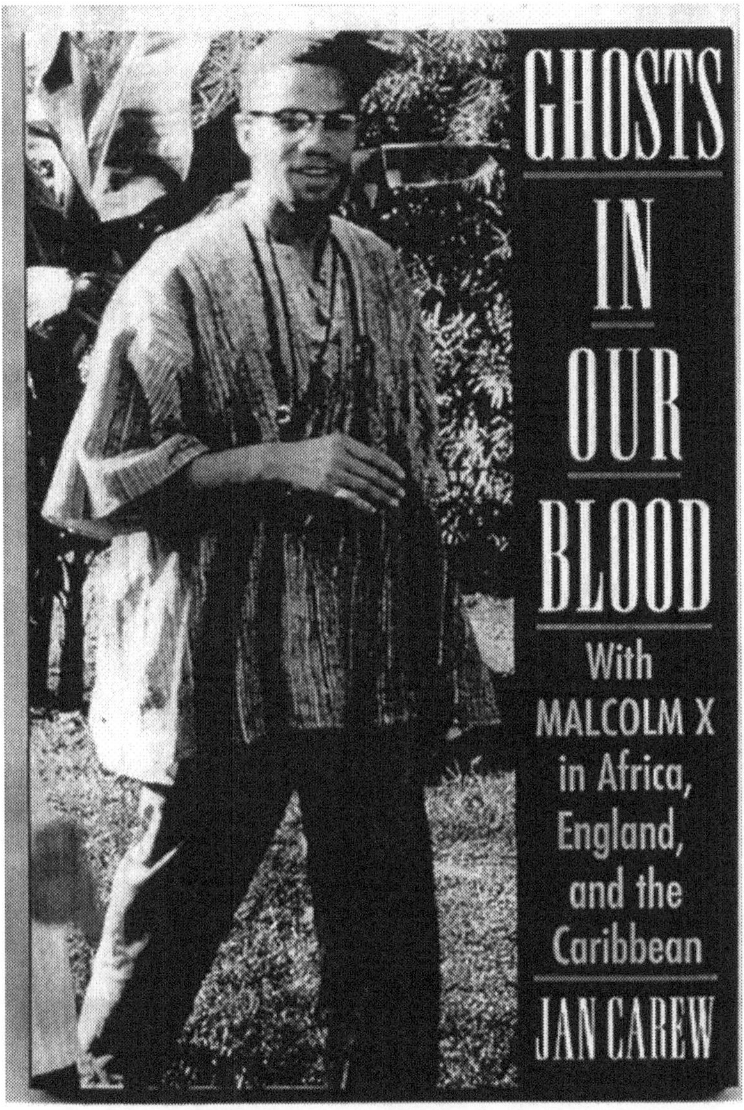
GHOSTS
IN
OUR
BLOOD
With
MALCOLM X
in Africa,
England,
and the
Caribbean
JAN CAREW

Preface

At the very beginning, allow me to make some points of clarification. It does not take long to discover through research that those hard-to-find early Chinese historical records are often conflicting in many ways. Much of the time, dates are only approximate and the names of old Chinese masters appear in many different spellings in English. Use of initial capital letters, hyphens, and apostrophes do not appear to follow any pattern of consistency and vowels often seem to be interchangeable. Many people experience confusion wondering if we are all talking about the same thing! Is it T'ai Chi or Tai Ch'i or Taiji? Should be Dai Ji or Daiji? Just when and how is it Chu'an, Chuan, or Quan? Why is it sometimes ch'i and at other times chi?[1]

T'ai Chi usually translates to mean supreme ultimate or grand ultimate or grand terminus while *Chu'an* and *Quan* usually mean boxing or fist. All of the spellings and forms are acceptable even though different forms of some words may carry slightly different meanings. I cannot even begin to explain the differences, but I can point out that they are generally attributable to variations in translating Chinese picture-characters into words. In addition to commonly accepted transliterations, there are two official systems of spelling in use. One is the ***Wade-Giles*** system developed in the Western tradition by two British linguists in the 19th century and the other is the ***Pinyin*** system developed by the Chinese themselves in Mainland China beginning in 1958. Therefore, in the Wade-Giles translation it is "T'ai Chi Ch'uan" while "Taijiquan" is the Pinyin translation. Much of the confusion comes from the interchange of words between these two systems of spelling and phonetics and is applicable to the whole discussion regarding the art. The names of people, places, and methods throughout the history of Taijiquan have many spelling variations in the written literature. Here,

---

1 *Ch'i* or *qi or ji* (pronounced "chee" and spelled "*chi*" throughout this book) is the Chinese word used to describe that intrinsic life energy or vital energy that exists in all living things.

for the sake of simplicity, I will drop all accent marks and consistently use "Tai Chi" while continuing to point out certain other instances where variations of words may be seen by the use of brackets—[ ]. Now that the easy part is out of the way, I will focus on the art of Tai Chi itself.

It is not my intention to promote Tai Chi as if it is an instant health cure or a short course in self-defense. This book is more of a reference for *why* to get started in Tai Chi than a manual of *how* to get started. Tai Chi is an art and, like all arts, time and diligent practice are required in order to perfect it. However, for those willing to persevere, the potential benefits can change a person's life altogether because they are not decreased by old age; in fact, there are many around the world who are still teaching Tai Chi well into their eighties.

> **t'ai chi ch'uan**
> *Pronunciation:* (tI' jE' chwän', chE'),
> a Chinese martial art and form of stylized, meditative exercise, characterized by methodically slow circular and stretching movements and positions of bodily balance. Also, **tai' chi' chuan'**; *Pinyin,* **tai ji quan**
> *Pronunciation:* (tI' jE' chyän'). Also called **t'ai' chi', tai' chi', tai' ji'.**

This is a simple enough dictionary definition to give to anyone in response to the question, "What is Tai Chi?" However, it is *my* intention to answer the question, "Why should *I* be interested in Tai Chi?" I am convinced that Tai Chi is the **ultimate** exercise for improving and maintaining good health long into our "golden" years. I have practiced the external martial arts for over forty years and have taught many students during that time, but I believe that the long-term benefits of Tai Chi for the practitioner far outweigh any of those systems.

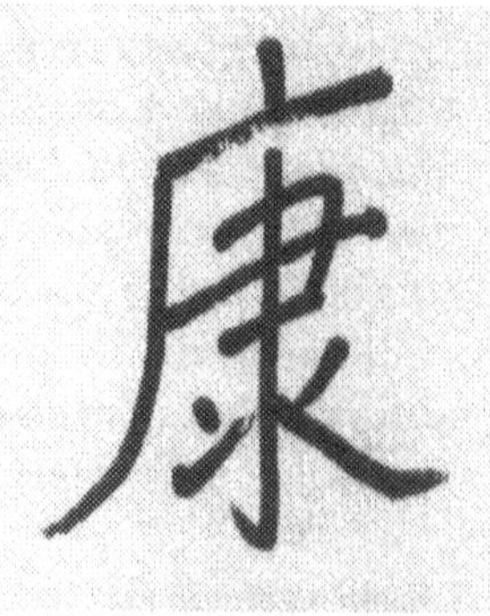

Tai Chi Healing Symbol

Tai Chi is an ancient martial and healing art. Although Tai Chi is not the only art of its kind, it is, by far, the most well known worldwide. Indeed, I believe that the world owes a debt of gratitude to the Chinese culture for preserving it through the years. Historically, it seems that using movement systems for health based on philosophy is part of the Eastern culture. Most of these systems include a martial application as well. In China alone, well over 300 different known martial arts styles exist. Of the popular modern styles of Tai Chi, some come, via various lineages, from noted masters of the art and reflect their personal expression of the system that they learned. Other styles come from those who have created new movement sequences for themselves and their students. Some of the forms are specifically for competition or general health care. No matter which style or form one practices, all Tai Chi is good Tai Chi as long as the traditional principles of the art are in tact. The goal of Tai Chi is to develop a more connected relationship between the practitioner's body, mind and spirit. Tai Chi is a particular type of *Kung Fu*, which means skill, ability, or work, generally applied to a rigorous martial art system of defense. These defense systems are characterized by open-hand techniques using slower, softer movements to circulate internal energy throughout the body. What makes this method of self-defense more useful is that it stresses overcoming external techniques using calmness and appropriate action. Because of its focus on internal energy, Tai Chi goes beyond its original martial arts intent. Initially, it may have been a fighting form, emphasizing strength, balance, flexibility, and speed. Through time, it has evolved into a soft, slow, and gentle form of exercise that people of all ages practiced. In Chinese tradition, there are thousands of methods and practices for self-healing generally called *Qigong*, also called *Chi Kung* or *Chi Gung*. Tai Chi, most often classified as an internal martial art, is one method of *Qigong*. This is a system of exercises to enhance health and vitality determined in accordance with the four pillars of Traditional Chinese Medicine (TCM): 1) looking at the facial color, the skin, the tongue; 2) smelling the breath, the body odor; 3) palpation, as in feeling the wrist pulse; 4) and listening to the patient's symptoms as well as the tone of the voice or the sound of a cough. Dedicated practice of Tai Chi has an effect on the body that can be visibly observed. Another effect of Tai Chi, balance or harmony, is summed up in the familiar symbol associated with the art.

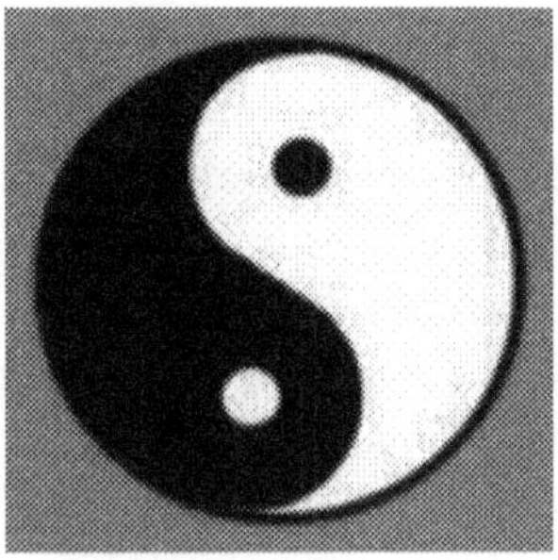

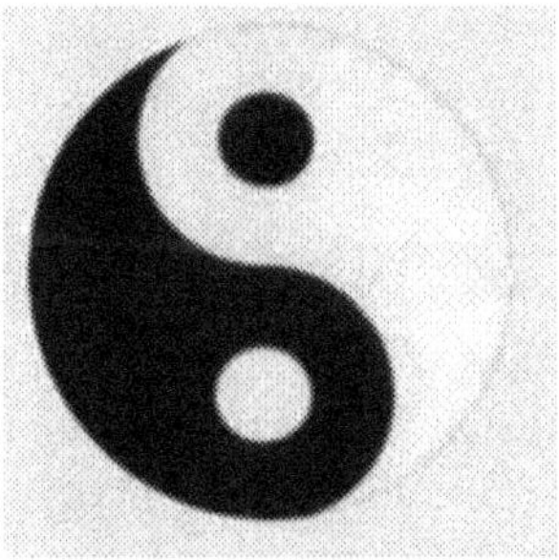

The Tai Chi symbol, depicting *Yin* and *Yang*, represents the ***ultimate*** to be achieved. One important thing to notice about *Yin* and *Yang* is that they only exist in relation to each other. In the symbol, two semicircles of dark (*Yin*) and light (*Yang*) make a complete circle as they constantly merge into each other portraying the harmony of motion. The written Chinese symbol for *Yin* is the dark side of the hill and that for *Yang* is the sunny side of the hill. The description of the Tai Chi symbol is often the "double fish" where the black areas represent *Yin* and the white areas represent *Yang*. The white fish has a black eye; the black fish has a white eye. This represents that both energies contain the potential for their opposite within them, such as a body moving through the Tai Chi form has a mind that is still. There are variations of this symbol but I use the one found in early texts of the Yang Family as the orientation for my Tai Chi classes. It is the symbol with the white fish on the top and right while the black fish is below and left, representing the ascending nature of *Yang* and the descending nature of *Yin*. No matter which orientation is used, the symbol describes the laws of *Yin* and *Yang*, which assert that all existence is a relationship between complimentary but opposing pairs. This polarity gives each part a seed of the other within it. In this system, *Yang* represent all that is expressive, productive and strength-oriented while its opposite, *Yin*, is receptive, yielding and internal. It is important not to attach 'good' and 'bad' labels to these qualities. In Chinese culture, balance and appropriate behavior are most important. The harmonious change from yielding to unbending happens in the form of a circle and the main pattern of Tai Chi is many circles spiraling continually without end. The philosophy and heritage of traditional Tai Chi span thousands of years. The Chinese discovered that the abilities of the human body are capable of development beyond their commonly perceived potential. One could reach the ultimate level, or develop in that direction, by means of balancing these two equal and complementary powers and their natural motions. Through moderation and natural living, the interaction of *Yin* and *Yang* produces harmony and brings unlimited development of the individual. The old masters of Tai Chi practiced justice, charity, the medicinal arts, and championed education as part of their lifestyle. Society-at-large adopted these codes for human conduct and everyone obeyed them; their enforcement was as strict as written laws.

Traditionally, Tai Chi principles passed down by word of mouth from generation to generation with much of the material handed down in legends and folk art. Traditional instruction occurred in a temple or the home of the master. It is only in recent years that the secret, temple form of the various styles became available to everyone and thereby escaped extinction. However, the more popular public styles are still quite beneficial and easily accessible as people continue to search for the ultimate—a peaceful and natural way of living. Tai Chi applies the idea of a natural harmony to the development of mind and body in a progressive, organized manner. Historically, followers of Tai Chi believed people should: 1) discipline themselves to be spiritual, healthy, kind and intelligent; 2) be responsible in assisting others to reach the same levels of achievement; 3) enjoy truth; 4) fight fearlessly against immorality and injustice; and 5) protect the needy and weak. This is because the bases of Tai Chi are the principles of the Tao [Dao]. While

Taoism [Daoism] is a system of profound philosophical thought that studies the earth, heavens, and nature, it also teaches the ideas of leading a secluded and quiet life, creating a tradition wherein one does not seek powerful positions and excesses, and contributing to the common good.

Tai Chi often receives criticism as a martial art because of its softness and relaxed, natural postures. These postures directly reflect the inseparable relationship between Taoism and Tai Chi. Many have observed only the public form of the art that developed apart from the need for defense. The public form of Tai Chi, originally developed to protect the secrets of the temple form used for defense, became the form taught for exercise and health. The ability to perform explosive whipping or snake-like striking from any position remains a secret trademark of all forms of Tai Chi. When practiced as a martial art, Tai Chi uses the mind to project the body's vital chi for higher-level, intricate, acupuncture-point striking ***without*** physical contact! Although this is one of the main reasons that Tai Chi as a martial art has been shrouded in mystery and secrecy and appears ineffective as a combat art, only a few practitioners achieve this level of mastery after many, many years. Tai Chi became the most powerful known martial art yielding awesome results in terms of human abilities coming from the power of the mind because of the legendary achievements of a few masters. Effort, concentration and dedication are required to attain even a fair level of achievement. This internal work involved is what makes the practice of Tai Chi the "grand ultimate" of all the martial arts. The majority of those practicing Tai Chi today do so to develop the *chi* to maintain and regenerate good health. Undeniably, Tai Chi with its flowing rhythm has the power of evoking this strong sensory response or *chi*. In Chapter 9 of this book, I list the correlation between some specific movements and the health of various parts of the body as the *chi* moves along the bioelectrical conduits or *meridians* of the body.

Customarily, the knowledge of the history of Tai Chi has been within the Chinese culture and the world considers it as a Chinese martial art. Therefore, as a "westerner" with a lack of knowledge of the language, customs and national developments in China, some barriers to fully comprehending the culture from which the modern art of Tai Chi emerged may be present. It is not only the variations of spelling and punctuation but also the different family styles of Tai Chi broken down into an endless number of forms along various lineages that only worsens the confusion.

This book represents the result of compiling information for my Tai Chi classes. The questions and topics covered a wide range but they were necessary to help my students embrace Tai Chi more fully. Therefore, while it may be true that each of the chapters of this book could stand apart from the others, it is my aim to give comprehensive background information about why the daily, systematic practice of Tai Chi is a wise and prudent choice for **YOU**. After that, instruction and discipline in the art is not only readily available but also more fully appreciated. First, endure the roll call of names, dates and places. It is important to understand some of the history of the art in order for you to join the continued practice of it because of the benefits it offers the human body. Discover with me the intrigue of Tai Chi and its relevance for you as an individual.

Then, it is my hope that this book not only reaches the masses that may yet still be unfamiliar with Tai Chi but also inspires each person to investigate further the daily practice of this amazing art.

Mfundishi Obuabasa Serikali
Louisville, Kentucky
April 2006

Acknowledgements

I sincerely thank Kumasi, Kitabu, and Khalilah, for their work to make this book a reality. Without their support, it certainly would not have been possible. Their talent for research, illustration, and organization made the project attainable. Kumasi is an angel put on this Earth to awaken the beauty and love within us through her writing. I feel truly blessed to walk with this angel incarnate.

I wish to give special acknowledgement to my mother, Mrs. Lenora Cowan and my grandmother, "Big Mama" (Matilda). I often reflect on their teachings from early in life as I continue to study.

Thanks to Dr. Mahn Saing for all of his advice and expertise.

I am grateful to Mr. Fred Simmons of Tuskegee, Alabama who died at the approximate age of 110 in 2002. "Uncle Fred", as he was known, imparted to me some of the timeless wisdom I have come to expect from the elders and that I try to pass on to others.

I give honorable mention to Mrs. Ada Lee Hosley, also in Tuskegee, who I count among my biggest fans. At the time of this writing, "Mama Ada" is 93 years young. Since I cannot do an adequate roll call of the countless seniors with whom I have shared time and laughter, she represents each of them.

There are many others who have encouraged me through the years whose names are too numerous to recount here. I am thankful for the energy and positive motivation I received from each of them.

Finally, I make the following acknowledgements for the photographs, artwork, and illustrations used in this endeavor:

- Cover Art graphic: *African and Chinese Monks Training*, Courtesy of Nijart International

- Dr. Jan Carew graphics (Preface): Courtesy of Dr. Jan Carew
- Li Tieguai graphic (Chapter 3): Courtesy of Gregory Smits, *Later Daoism* (www.east-asian-history.net/textbooks/PM-China/Ch7/18.jpg) from the web-based book *Topics in Pre-Modern China History* (www.east-asian-history.net/textbooks/PM-China)
- Chapter 7 Illustrations: Taheeda Kumasi Serikali
- All other photographs: Property of the author unless otherwise noted
- All other illustrations: Public domain clipart

The greatest gift you have to give the world is that of your own self-transformation.

-Lao Tzu (Hua Hu Ching, chapter 75)

1

Tai Chi and Mfundishi Obuabasa Serikali

Welcome to a world filled with love! It is the world of healing and meditative movements. This book attempts to capture decades of work and healing within the montage of vibration movements known as Tai Chi. These movements exist to create physical, emotional and mental wholeness. Tai Chi is a journey that takes us from the beginning to the end of the day on the planet Earth. If every day is the beginning of a new life and an awakening, let it be the love energy of all that is that empowers and motivates. Through love, we can unite and heal this planet, one heart at a time, and ourselves. My present work with Tai Chi rests on the foundation of my lifelong interest in the martial arts. I do not wish to write this book without recalling the path that I have traveled.

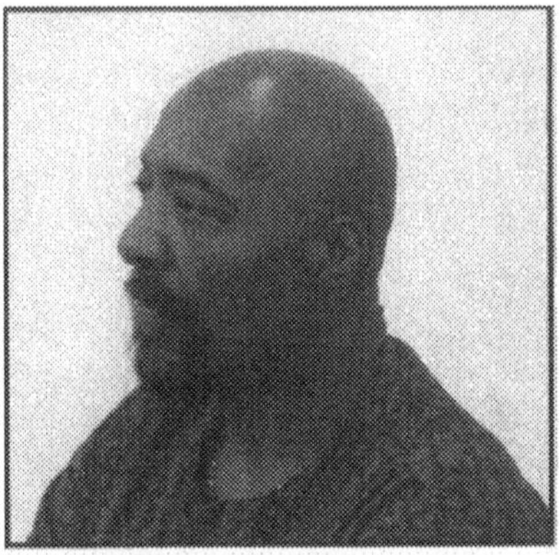

Born G. C. Cowan, Jr. in Louisville, Kentucky in 1941, the second son of Mrs. and Mrs. George (Lenora) Cowan, I began as a student of the martial arts over 40 years ago. My interest developed early when, at age 15, I ordered a book, *The Way of Karate,* by Bruce Tiger and began my self-taught studying and practicing. After high school, while away at New Mexico Highlands University I began training with a Japanese foreign exchange student in the art of *Shotokan* Karate. Upon returning home, I found other brothers who had received training during their military service and we began training together. Shortly thereafter, I began my formal martial arts training at the Louisville Fall City Judo School under Earl Cheatham, another ex-military martial artist who trained at the *Kotokan* School in Japan. As a result, I received my first black belt in Judo from the Grandmaster of the *Kotokan* School during his visit to Louisville.

I formed relationships with several other brothers, such as Grandmaster Lloyd Johnson and the late Grandmaster Dana Matthewson, who were on this same journey of discovery through the martial arts. I consider another of these men, Grandmaster Henry Cook, to be a martial arts genius. He is the founder of the Kumasi African Stick Fighting System and continues to teach and train students today. The school we established during that time served as a central point for other black men seeking an outlet for growth. This was during turbulent times in the city and our school became a gathering place for the brothers in the struggle for the rights of black people. As the school became popular, I served as a teacher of martial arts for such programs and organizations as Nation of Islam, Black Panther Party, JOMO Revolutionary Party, Black African Congress, Pan-African Liberation Party, NAACP, and the Urban League. The Fruit of Islam asked me to do martial arts training, which led to serving as a bodyguard for many entertainers and dignitaries who came to Louisville. Our school received much recognition and earned many awards. Eventually, as the course of social action for black people changed, I felt that egos began to grow bigger than the art, larger than the school, greater than the culture, more important than unity, and more profitable than brotherhood. Profit was the main keyword and brotherhood, unity, culture and art all fell to it. I wanted to seek the art and began on the next part of my journey that led me to Chicago.

In Chicago, I was introduced to Otis and Preston Baker of the Baker Dojo where I found art, culture, unity and brotherhood once more. This was a turning point in my life where I dedicated myself to the art and to the Black Power movement. Here I formed some of the closest relationships I have ever had with other black men—relationships and love that continue today. Men like Brad Hughes, "Shorty" Mills, and "Jaco" became like a second family to me as well as worthy opponents. The fight I fought against Jaco, a gentle giant, was one of the greatest fights of my life. My training with the Baker brothers strengthened my standing in the martial arts community across the nation. I won many championships and received numerous awards and accolades. Through the Chicago school I met many warriors and legends such as Ben Peacock, Moses Powell, Kalinde Iye, Grandmaster Jimmy Jones, and Baba Vita. The training and teaching I had already received from JaJa Uthman and Robert "Capri" Hawkins, cultural mentors, inspired me to seek out and live by African culture.

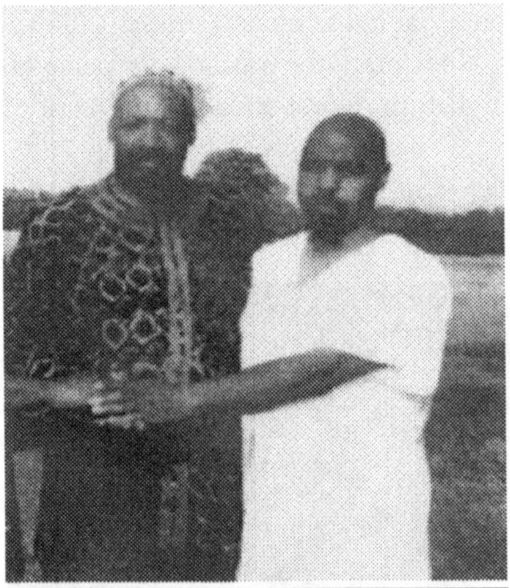

Mfundishi Obuabasa Serikali and Nganga Mfundish Tolo-Naa

During the time spent in Chicago, I met two brothers who helped me along this path. I studied with Nganga Mfundishi Tolo-Naa (formerly known as RaymondCooper) for over 20 years. Nganga Mfundishi Tolo-Naa began studying martial arts at the age of twelve. Throughout the mid-1960s, he competed successfully in Karate tournaments in the United States and Canada. In 1964, he took second place in the World Karate Championship. He has studied a broad range of martial arts including Jiu jitsu, Judo, Karate, Tae kwon do, Akido, Shao lin, Bando, Tai Chi Chuan, Hsing-yi Chuan, Pa-Kua Chang, and many long and short weapon routines. He is the originator of the Shackle Hand Style of self-defense. He is a student of many meditative disciplines including Taoist Yoga, Kundalini Yoga, Tantra Yoga, and Hatha Yoga. He received his initiation in Tibetan Tantra meditation from His Holiness the Dalai Lama. Over the past 30 years, Nganga Mfundishi Tolo-Naa has concentrated on the study of Chinese internal systems with the late Professor Huo Chi-Kwang[2] and the late Grandmaster Lu Hung-Ping[3]. In the 1960s, Nganga Mfundishi Tolo-Naa founded the All-African People's Art and Cultural Center. In the 1980s, he started the *Maat Center for Martial Arts* in Chicago Heights. Besides being a

2 Professor Huo Chi-Kwang was born in the Hopei province of China. He was a master of calligraphy, painting, and poetry as well as a master boxer. During World War II, Professor Huo was president of the National Oriental Languages College in China. Professor Huo had complete training in the Chinese physical disciplines. He studied Tai Chi Chuan and was the third generation of Pa-Kua Chuan masters tracing his instructor lineage back to a hermit monk who refused the usage of his name. In Taipei in 1965, Professor Huo co-founded the Tai Chi Chuan Learning Society. After arriving in Chicago over thirty years ago, he founded the Chinese Cultural Academy in Evanston (Ill.) and was the first to teach Tai Chi Chuan in the Chicago area. Professor Huo was in his early nineties when he died in January 1998.

legendary martial artist and a traditional herbal healer, he is co-founder of the Kupigana Ngumi Martial Arts Federation and founder of the Martial Arts Research Society. *Kupigana Ngumi* is a fighting style meaning "Way of Fighting with the Fist." In 1987, he founded QuieScience Sacred Science Temple (QSST), a not-for-profit, non-religious organization dedicated to promoting personal development through the martial arts. Through him, I met Mfundishi Maasi of New York.

Shaha Mfundishi Maasi (formerly known as William Nichols, Jr.) developed an early interest in martial science and began his formal training in 1959 while serving in the U.S.M.C. Upon transferring to Kaneohe Bay, Hawaii in the early 1960's, he studied *Kempo* under Staff Sergeant Robert Holt of American Samoa. After his discharge in 1962, Maasi studied under the legendary combat master James Cheatham in Newark, New Jersey. At the death of Master Cheatham, Maasi established his first school located in Newark, which he later closed to began study under Dr. U Maung Gyi, the father of *Bando* in America. Shaha Mfundishi Maasi was the first non-Burmese to attain the "third level of enlightenment" and the title Saya (teacher) under Dr. Gyi. After his introduction to the Burmese Monk System of meditation and self-defense, Maasi attained the fourth level of achievement from the International and American Bando Association. The work of Maasi, along with Nganga Mfundishi Tolo-Naa, culminated in the founding of the African warrior style of *Kupigana Ngumi.* His early efforts to establish that the roots of martial science originated in Egypt gained the

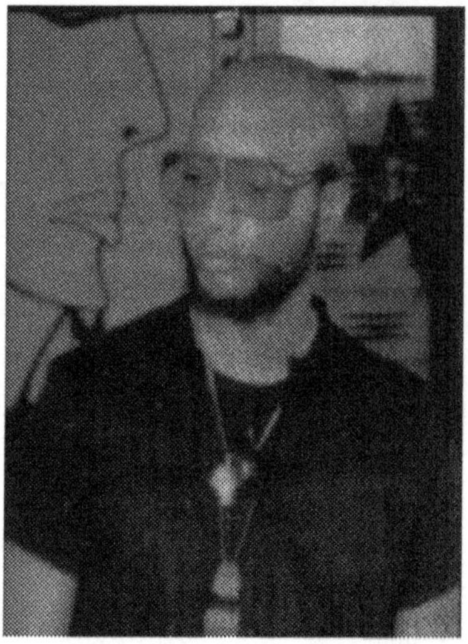

Shaha Mfundishi Maasi

[3] Grandmaster Lu Hung-Ping was a renowned internal arts master and teacher. He taught in Chicago from 1987 until his death in 1990, at the age of 91. Although Grandmaster Lu was an authority on his specialty, Pa-Kua Chuan, he was well versed in all the traditional Chinese martial arts. At the age of 30, Grandmaster Lu opened the first school for Pa-Kua and Hsing-yi Chuan in China where he only taught other masters. In his later years, he traveled and taught his belief in Tai Chi Chuan as a way of life and as a way to achieve and maintain health, harmony, and balance within oneself and the world.

support of Grandmaster Dr. Gyi (Burmese) and Grandmaster Alan Lee (Chinese). Because of his studies of African spiritual traditions and fighting arts and his dedication to the Pan African struggle, Dr. Maulana Karenga conferred upon him the title "Mfundishi" (Grandmaster) and empowered him to confer that title upon others under his training. In addition, Maasi has also studied Jiu-Jitsu, Karate, Yoga, Kuo Shu, Tai-Ki-Ken, Tai Chi Chuan, Hsing I Chuan, Tai Chi Ruler, and a wide variety of the weaponry of Africa and Asia. Maasi has also served as a Non-governmental Organizational Representative to the United Nations for the Congress of African People, Royal Retainer to His Majesty Nana Kablam I of Azzureti Village (Grand Bassam, Cote d'Ivoire, West Africa), and a delegate to the 7th Pan African Congress (Kampala, Uganda, East Africa). Shaha Mfundishi Maasi continues to present the higher principles of the African Warrior tradition and *Kupigana Ngumi* throughout the diaspora through teaching and lecturing.

Although I was born and raised in these United States, I long ago decided to emulate the ways of my ancestors and teach those ways to others in whatever form of the arts I engaged. Professor Asa Hilliard wrote an article titled *To Be an African Teacher* in which he wrote the following:

> *African teachers focus the curriculum on the real and the true, on what was, what is, and on what can be, in keeping with divine principles. African teachers place a premium on bringing their students into a knowledge of themselves and a knowledge of their communities. African people place great value on WHO each person is, on WHO the community is and the honored place that each member of the family occupies within the community. African teachers respect mastery, and seek through apprenticeship to learn from true masters, masters who are valued agents of the African community, who are steeped in the deep thought and behavior of the community, who exhibit an abiding unshakable primary loyalty to the community and who are in constant communication with the wise elders of the community. African teachers recognize the genius and the divinity of each of our children, speaking to and teaching to each child's intellect, humanity, and spirit. We do not question a child's possession of these things. In touching the intellect, humanity and spirit within children, African teachers recognize the centrality of relationships between teachers and students, among students, and within the African community as a whole. For the African teacher, teaching is a calling, a constant journey towards mastery, a scientific activity, a matter of community membership, an aspect of a learning community, a process of "becoming a library," a*

> *matter of care and custody for our culture and traditions, a matter of a critical viewing of the wider world, and a response to the imperative of MAAT. The African teacher is a parent, friend, guide, coach, healer, counselor, model, storyteller, entertainer, artist, architect, builder, minister, and advocate to and for students. Typically the African teacher leads a social collective process, one where social bonds are reinforced or created. In this social process, the destinies of the students are connected to each other, to their families, to their communities, to their ancestors, to those who are yet to be born, to their environment, to their traditions, to MAAT as a way of life, and to their Creator.*

My spiritual journey of this period led me to Ohio where I first saw the art of Tai Chi performed in a camp of the Bhagwan Shree Rajneesh. I also spent time in the Hare Krishna community where I studied the principles of Yoga. However, I must credit my spiritual training to my grandmother, Big Mama (Matilda), a Mississippi Red Dirt Choctaw Indian. She was a praying woman who had the gift of healing. She was also a master herbalist and midwife and she trained me well to observe, be still and seek to know myself. From Big Mama's training, I found what I know today to be "Christ Consciousness." It has kept me from becoming a part of today's 'medicated' society. Instead, I continue to want to be a seeker of life like Big Mama, one who yielded to the forces of nature and love. I have remembered all that she taught me, not only about herbs and nature, but also about life and people:

> *It is not what people owe me that is important; it is what I owe others that is.*
> *God owes me nothing; I owe my Creator everything.*
> *This world owes me nothing; I owe the world everything.*
> *My enemies owe me nothing; I owe my enemies everything.*

After my return to Louisville, I founded several Karate schools and taught many students. My teams and I fought in tournaments in many places, including Chicago, and brought many sweet victories back to Louisville during the 1970s. Over the next two decades, the demand for Karate training remained high and I invested my time and energy in training young men and women in the discipline of the martial arts through it. Eventually, my interest moved away from the high energy of the youth of the community toward the mature adults of the community. One day, while engaged in my Tai Chi routine on a pleasant day in the park, I attracted a few onlookers wanting to know more about this exercise. I asked them to join me and that was the beginning of my next level of involvement with the community through martial arts.

I hold memberships in several national and international Tai Chi organizations, including the International Yang Style Tai Chi Chuan Association, but my work and effort in them is minimal. Most recently, I obtained membership in the American Yangjia Michuan Tajiquan Association (AYMTA). Currently, the International Tai Chi Alliance certifies me as a Tai Chi instructor. In this capacity, I conduct *Movements for Health (MFH)* classes through the Metro Louisville (Kentucky) Health Department as part of the *Mayor's Healthy Hometown Movement*. This honor is a direct result of classes for seniors begun several years ago. To date, hundreds have been introduced to the art of Tai Chi and have added Tai Chi to their regimen for health and longevity. I am firmly committed to helping others realize their maximum potential, regardless of age. The reward for me is seeing people who were not previously involved in any physical activity living a more healthy, happy and abundant life.

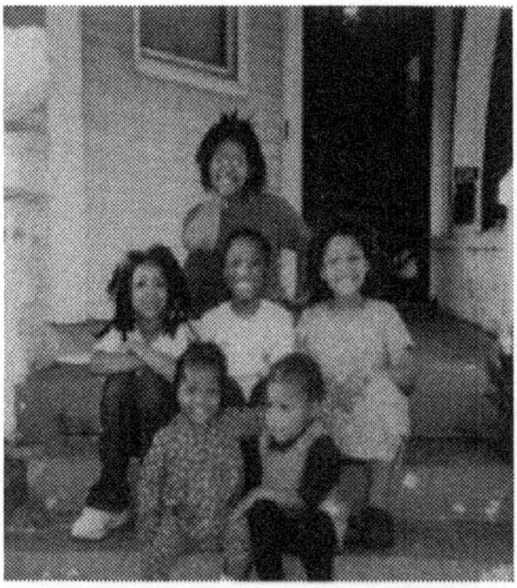

Tai Chi future—
1st row: Indigo, Aaliyah;
2nd row: Ajahla, Kyanna, Mesa;
Top: Obi Nana (2002)

As Tai Chi begins with intent, I also write this book with intent—not to disparage any, but to enlighten some. It is not my intent to promote a 'new' way, but rather to remind concerning that which we already know. I am not a master of Tai Chi. I have no desire for a 'following' of my own; instead, it is my intent that we all should follow the precepts of good health and a sound mind through wisdom. I have had the good fortune of being in the company of many well-know individuals. Throughout the years and regardless of the achievements, I continue to devote my life to a quest for higher consciousness, pan-African empowerment, and unity of the masses. I intend to continue to teach in the tradition of Bodhidharma: promoting Tai Chi for improved health, increased strength, spiritual meditation focused on love of self, others and God, and mental stillness and calmness within the individual. I see the future of Tai Chi for my people in the faces of my children. I hope that each of them not only embraces the art but also passes it on as needed medicine. My fellow angels, our time together is a precious journey in which all of us agreed to different paths and experiences. Many of us have chosen to stay connected unconsciously one way or another through relationships, work, or even a passing glance from a stranger who looked familiar.

The movement and breath used in the art of Tai Chi unite us all for a few moments in time. Let us awaken the power of love within us and learn to share this love. We are all connected.

My opponent's strength merely brushed my skin, but my will power has penetrated into his bones.

~Master Li Yi Yu

2

Tai Chi Traditional History

Chinese history has mentioned breathing and inner *chi* energy since around 800 BC. Hau Tuo [Hau To], a famous Taoist physician of the Han Dynasty and considered to be the father of Chinese surgery, practiced a system of exercises using deep breathing methods and movements that he claimed would extend one's longevity to over one hundred years. The exercises, aptly called 'frolics of five animals' or 'five animals play', were based on the movements of the tiger, deer, ape, bear, and bird. Hua Tuo's belief was that motion is fundamentally important to health and that by mimicking the movements of different animals; all parts of the body receive exercise and stretching, thereby activating the flow of fluid and energy in the body.

Among researchers and historians, the factual history of Tai Chi has many points of dissention laced throughout it. What exists today is more probably a mix between ancient history and myth. There are several versions of the origin of Tai Chi all of which converge at a point to bring us through to the modern development of the art. What follows is a composite version meant to give a brief overview of the colorful history of Tai Chi.

The legendary founder of Tai Chi was Chang San-feng [Zhang Zhan-feng], a Taoist monk of the Wu Tang Monastery [Wu Dong/Wu Dang/Wudang] at the end of the Sung Dynasty. He was born poor, a son of a farmer who loved martial arts and studied Shaolin *Hing Quan*. He began his spiritual journey as a Shaolin disciple, but supposedly left the temple because he thought that the fighting techniques developed there had become too harsh and brute strength oriented. He traveled to Wu Tang Mountain and spent many years there as a hermit observing the habits of animals such as turtles and cranes. It is said that he witnessed a fight between a large bird and a snake. According to legend, Chang was sitting one dawn observing his garden in quiet meditation. As the sun arose and began to shine, a snake crawled out upon one of the flat rocks to sun itself. A large bird sitting in a tree above the garden saw the snake and determined it was to be its dinner. The bird flew down from the tree, swooping down upon the snake with all the force it could muster from its high vantage point. The snake, using its sinuous and continuously flowing movements, transmitted the force of the bird to the rock and allowed the bird to dash itself upon the ground. Repeatedly, with each attack of the bird, the snake defended itself by yielding and allowing the force expended by the bird to turn against the attacker. Every time the bird spread its wings and attacked, the snake would move slightly to escape the attack, but maintained it usual coiled shape. This sparring contest continued for many hours, through which Chang recognized the value in circular movement and realized that soft wins over hard. Learning and adapting these natural movements to the mechanics of the human body and connecting them with the martial arts he already knew using the guiding principles of Taoism, Chang Sen-feng developed his Grand/Supreme Ultimate System of internal martial arts. He eventually returned to the Shaolin temple where he taught his new internal art often called Wu Tang Boxing [Wudang Internal Boxing]. His form consisted of *Thirteen Postures* (or Eight Gates and Five Attitudes) that corresponded to the eight primary trigrams of the *I Ching* and the five elements of the Tao in fundamental Chinese philosophy. The gates were eight postures that represented eight different types of strength: ward-off, rollback, press, push, pull, split or twist, elbow strike, shoulder strike. Additionally, the attitudes were the five different directions for the application of the gates: advance, retreat, look left, gaze right, central equilibrium. His exercises stressed suppleness and elasticity and were opposed to hardness and force while incorporating philosophy, physiology, psychology, geometry and the laws of dynamics.

Chang Sung-chi was a student of Chang Sen-feng who passed the *Thirteen Postures* on to his student, Wang Chung-yeuh, who is responsible for joining the movements into a continuous flow. Subsequently Wang Chung-yeuh's student, Chiang Fa [Jiang Fa] taught in a village of Wen County, Honan Province known as Chenjiagon Village as "Chen" was the surname of most of its inhabitants. From this beginning in the Chen family, several lines of Tai Chi developed through four disciples of Chiang Fa: Chen You-heng, Chen Chang-hsing, Chen Yau-pin, and Chen Wang Ting.

At this point in the history of the development of Tai Chi, the lines of succession multiply immensely through replication and discovery. The Chinese, in isolation from the rest of the world, practiced the art of Tai Chi for many years and the techniques remained a secret under the Chen dynasty. During the early 1800s, these techniques were passed to those outside of the Chen family via Yang Lu Chan and eventually were taught openly to the public. Later, during the 1930s, the knowledge of Tai Chi was greatly advanced outside of China through the efforts of the Yang family. Yang Cheng Fu, son of Yang Chien Hou and grandson of Yang Lu Chan determined to spread the knowledge of Tai Chi to the masses and further developed the slow, even-paced style that is characterized by large leaning movements and ward-off energy.

The 1960s brought about a time known as 'The Chinese Cultural Revolution' in Chinese history. Among other things, all intellectual or spiritual forms of *Qigong* became crimes against the "people" thereby outlawing the people's practice of Tai Chi as well. During this time when many Tai Chi masters actually fled China to teach elsewhere, the introduction of Tai Chi outside of China fostered the spread of Tai Chi around the world. (It was during this period of the 1960s that Cheng Man-Ching [Zheng Manqing], one of the greatest masters of his time, introduced Tai Chi to the United States.) After this era in history, China reclaimed certain aspects of her ancient tradition. For a short period of time, Tai Chi, usually Yang Style, was actually the only "party certified" system of health enhancement allowed. As it became clear that many forms of *Qigong* were beneficial to people's health, the various forms of Tai Chi also re-emerged. While China opened up to the world in general, interest in the Chinese arts significantly increased in direct proportion to the world's involvement with China. Western science became more open towards eastern science after witnessing the success of acupuncture and acupressure techniques, both of which increased interest in this eastern idea of *chi*.

Cheng Man-Ching, also known as Professor Cheng Man-Ching or Great Grandmaster Cheng Man-Ching, was a top disciple of Yang Lu-Chan's grandson, Yang Cheng-Fu, and was instrumental in popularizing Tai Chi and making it more accessible. He shortened the Yang style form, with his master's permission, to 37 postures to focus on the most important movements and eliminate some repetition making it the most popular of all the forms practiced. This form is characterized by its upright spine, rollback energy, and softness. Cheng traveled to the United States to teach and his students represented all backgrounds, explaining why the Yang form is so popular here today. Cheng Man-Ching taught American students at his studio in New York City, until his death in

1975. Fortunately, for the Chinese people, the Chinese government adopted Tai Chi as part of their public school curriculum ensuring the continuity of the legacy of the art within China. Today, foreign visitors to China can witness unimaginable crowds of people as they practice in the parks and open spaces early in the morning.

I will close this chapter by adding that there are those who contend that no one created Tai Chi. Their position is that Tai Chi is a combining of diverse conceptions of various systems of movement and meditation already practiced in China and that it evolved through the years into the coherent art form we have today. That, as they say, is another story for you, the reader, to investigate.

Yield and Overcome;
Bend and be straight.
Empty and be full...

-Lao Tzu (Tao Te Ching)

3

Tai Chi Familial Styles

Regardless of the origins of the Chinese culture, I had previously established the development of Tai Chi as it was passed through the Chen family of China for 200 years. All subsequent Tai Chi styles are derived from the original Chen family style and came to be associated with different families in China. These family names now designate the different styles of Tai Chi that have emerged. Each of the styles is arranged into sets of forms with different speeds, intensities, and amounts of physical power used. All contain similar sequences of movements that can be used for attack, defense, and health improvement. Of the numerous styles or families of Tai Chi, there are five that are practiced most commonly today.

From the early years of development of Tai Chi up to the present, the correct methods and techniques were secrets within the Tai Chi families. It was normal to "knock on the door" for at least a year before being accepted as a student by the senior masters. Within the traditional Tai Chi families, knowledge of the full secret techniques passed down carefully within the family or disciples. Even daughters could not learn the art because, should they marry, their husbands would have the family secrets. The **Chen Style** was no different and was not available to outsiders. The art occupied a place of such high esteem that not even anyone who had a bad disposition could be a student. This was the only way to ensure the authenticity and integrity of the form. The style was created using elements of Shaolin Cannon Pounding and Shaolin Red Fist resulting in fast, athletic movements and techniques for use in hand-to-hand combat. Its forms emphasize graceful, powerful, and explosive movements, as well as foot and fist actions. Many of the movements involve spinning and turning, and some sets include jumps and dodges. Present-day Chen style Tai Chi has refined these into two main sets, one with 83 postures and the other with 71 postures. A study from Beijing, China showed that practitioners of Chen style Tai Chi have faster reflexes than practitioners of other styles have. The fast and hard movements seem particularly beneficial to those people who need to expend energy quickly, or for those who need a more expressive emotional outlet.

According to legend, one day Yang Lu Chan [Yang Lu Tsan] witnessed a scene between a shop assistant and an unmanageable customer. The customer attacked the assistant, also a member of the Chen family, who dismissed him easily and sent him flying out the door of the shop. Yang Lu Chan was determined to learn the Chen family art and pestered the shop assistant for information. However, the assistant dutifully denied having any great knowledge himself but offered to recommend him to a great martial arts master in the Chen village. Since only Chen family members learned the art, the shop assistant wrote a letter recommending Yang Lu Chan as a servant to work for the family so that Yang Lu Chan could learn the art there. He earned his room and board and studied martial arts but could not learn the Chen martial arts. One night he accidentally stumbled upon a group practicing in the back courtyard. From that time on, he secretly began to observe and practice what he saw. Yang Lu Chan became so skilled from this clandestine instruction that he could correct the other students. Grandmaster Chen Chang Xin [Chen Chang-hsing] was so impressed by this that he broke family tradition and consented to teach Yang Lu Chan secretly to ensure the spread of the art outside of the Chen family.

The **Yang Style** evolved during the late 1800s after Yang Lu Chan modified the Chen style according to his previous martial arts training. After mastering the art through fourteen years of training, including two additional trips to the Chen village, Yang Lu Chan returned home where he taught martial arts for a living. His art was so soft and yielding that people first called it *mein quan* meaning cotton fist/boxing or *hua quan* meaning neutralizing fist/boxing. He was so skilled that he earned the nickname "Yang the Unsurpassed" and in all of his matches, no one was ever hurt. Later he moved to Beijing where he opened a school of Tai Chi and began teaching. It is here that many came to see his matches as his reputation soared. Also during this time, Ong Tong He, a Chinese scholar, witnessed his techniques and believed that they physically expressed the principles of Taiji (the philosophy). After that, Yang Lu Chan's art became known as Taijiquan and the various resulting styles took the same name.

In the Yang style, the *Thirteen Postures* received more emphasis than in the Chen style although the quick and explosive movements remained. Over time, the Yang style has been revised and softened, de-emphasizing the more forceful and difficult movements. Yang Lu Chan noticed that the Chen style was very difficult for the average practitioner to learn, so he modified it for health purposes and ease of flow. He softened the art developed by Chen Wang Ting, who was a disciple of Chiang Fa, by removing many of the more vigorous jumping tactics and feet stamping moves. In the present Yang style of Tai Chi, each movement flows seamlessly into the next one, as *Yin* flows into *Yang* and back into *Yin*. Inside each must remain an element of the other as the extremes draw near so the desire to return becomes greater creating the natural flowing oscillation that is the form. This is by far the most popular form of Tai Chi practiced today characterized by light, natural, and fully extended movements. It has three different forms: the simplified form, the short form, and the long form. The Yang lineage also resulted in three of the five most important schools of Tai Chi in existence today.

Yang Lu Chan and his second son, Yang Ban-ho [Yang Pan Hou], taught a set of movements called the *small style* in their surrounding area. A Manchurian guard at the imperial palace by the name of Quan Yu [also Wu Chan Yo or Wu Quan Yu] learned the style and taught it to his son, Wu Jianquan [also Wu Ching Chan or Wu Chien Chuan]. Quan Yu built upon the Chen style by adding throwing and grappling techniques while retaining its small, round movements. He gave attention to protecting one's body while retaining the soft natural characteristics. Wu Jianquan taught his interpretation of the Yang small style to others and it is today the **Wu Style**. This style contains more locking, pushing, and throwing techniques than the Yang style. It has slow and fast forms wherein the slow form does not include jumps or leaps, but rather emphasizes circular movements of the wrist and body while the fast form includes more flexible and swift movements.

Wu Yuxiang created the **Wu Shi Style** [also **Woo** or **Hao**] around 1852. He taught his nephew, Lee I-ye, who in turn taught Hao Wei-chen. Hao Wei-chen is responsible for removing some of the original high kicks and explosive movements. This style is a combination of the older Chen method learned from Yang Lu Chan and the newer style Chen method interpreted by Chen Quingping. It is a compact set emphasizing bodywork and exertion of the inner power. Wu Shi is very popular in China but is relatively unknown in the United States.

Hao Wei-chen later taught Wu Shi style to Sun Lu-tang who also studied Hsing-I Quan and Pa Kua Chang. Sun Lu-tang later made modifications in the Wu Shi style based on his past martial arts training resulting in the **Sun style**. Sun style

Tai Chi is very open allowing for the maximum flow of chi with emphasis on small stepping movements, small circular movements and high stances. It is a smooth style incorporating follow-up footwork, twisting and circular movements to build flexibility and agility. Sun style combined the strong points of Wu Shi style, Pa Kua Chang and Hsing-I Quan into a distinctive personal style. Sun style consists of three form sets: the high set, the low set and the fighting set. The use of the high set is mainly for relaxation and general health. The low set emphasizes strength and conditioning. The fighting set combines elements from the high and low sets to develop defense skills. The teaching of high set is open and without any restraints. The other two sets are secrets of the system, taught only to the most trusted students. Sun style is one of the less popular styles of Tai Chi.

The Chinese government recognizes these five family styles, which still find propagation through these lineage rights. There is a sixth style often mentioned: Zhao Bao. Chen Quin-ping, a student of Chen Yau-pun who was a student of Chiang-Fa, apparently developed this style. There are many styles of Tai Chi taught and described as "based on" one of the family styles—all of which go back to Chen style through the Yang style somehow. The circumstances have now changed a great deal and there is no longer any great need for secrecy with the patriarchal barriers mostly removed. However, some instructors and masters still refuse to teach openly. Some of the more popular forms practiced today were developed by the Chinese government to promote the art both as a form of health exercise and as a sport beginning in 1956. These national forms were taught to the masses and do not stress the martial aspects of the art. With the adoption of Wushu as an Olympic demonstration sport, the Chinese government has also increased the promotion of competition Tai Chi routines. There is one shortened routine for each major style of Tai Chi. There are also forms that combine aspects of all the different styles using selected techniques representative of the parent styles. Before 1988, it was difficult to evaluate Tai Chi routines because there was not any standard. Because of this, the 11th Asian Games in 1990 first saw the newly created 42-Form competition style. This choreographed style involves a high degree of difficulty and is a combination of the main characteristics of four major Tai Chi styles (Chen, Yang, Sun, and Wu). Because of the official recognition by the Chinese government and the Olympic Council, these forms have become the choice for many who simply want to enhance their health.

Various teachers and students have continued to teach their interpretations and modifications of the traditional movements just as in China those who learned the modified version as taught by Yang Lu Chan to the Manchu guards and the Imperial Family also continued to teach as a direct student of the master. The differences among the many schools of Tai Chi may or may not be evident. There may be hundreds of varieties of forms differing in postures or repetitions of postures. All of the styles are "systems" meaning that the solo forms are only one part of an entire system designed for combat. During the times of great political turmoil and upheaval in China efforts were made to preserve as much of the art as possible. I have already alluded to how Yang Lu Chan changed the form he taught at the palace to emphasize its health-giving benefit and de-emphasize its secret combat use. In order to keep the knowledge to a select few, the teaching of the weapons or combat training techniques was not open. I believe that, although preservation of the knowledge of the entire art was essential, a new consciousness that moved away from combative aggression and defensiveness developed in the East. For instance, in Japan the Japanese *'-jutsu'* fighting methods such as kenjutsu, jujutsu, aikijutsu, etc. were converted into the path of self-development or *'-do'* ways of kendo, judo, and aikido. However, the West needed shorter, more attainable forms due to the highly hurried way of life. Both paths are reasons for the proliferation of Tai Chi students worldwide who seek calmness and relaxation. In the solo form performed today, the opponent is unseen and may very well be "self." This is, perhaps, another reason why Tai Chi is sometimes called "shadow boxing." Imagine the solo Tai Chi practitioner in a battle with his/her own ego—the grand ultimate is total self-control. Just as *Yin* and *Yang* are infinite, so the ultimate can never be achieved—only approached. Because it is possible to become so very absorbed, I sometimes call it "spirit dancing" as well.

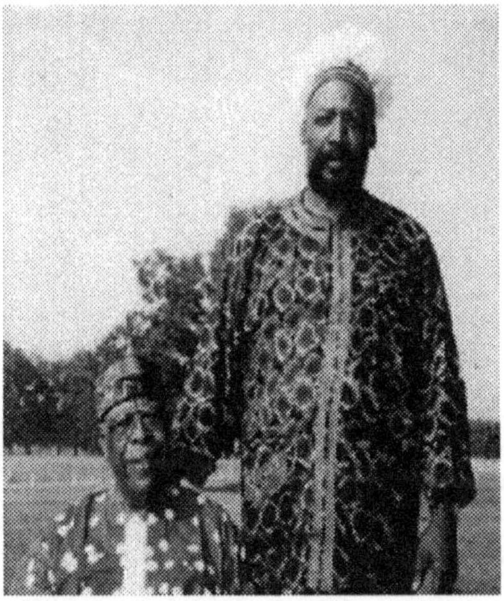

Mfundishi Serikali and teacher, Olowu Kunle

The quality of lineage continues to be a dominating factor in learning Tai Chi as with other martial arts. If a student had a good teacher who learned from a good teacher, then that person matures in the art as well. It is important to know a teacher's lineage and those who have verifiable lineages do not hesitate to make them known. I have chosen the 24-posture Yang short form as the style of Tai Chi I practice and teach. This is primarily due to the availability of this form to me at the time I began to earnestly study Tai Chi. With the rapid development of Tai Chi in this country, I wanted to teach that which was most familiar yet according to the basic tenets and principles of Tai Chi.

The first brother to teach me to the art of Tai Chi was Nganga Mfundishi Tolo-Naa in 1976. He is from a very distinguished lineage that also became my lineage through him. Since that time, I have had many teachers including books, videos, seminars and workshops. I am not a master of Tai Chi but a practitioner or player. To this day, I remain a student to other players who have something to share on the subject of Tai Chi.

In contrast, the love of wisdom in the ancient civilizations of Egypt, India, and China was a living dynamic process. That which we refer to as philosophy comprised the guidelines to which they intellectually adhered. But their ever present reality was that true transformation is not possible through development of the intellect alone, regardless of the amount of information consumed. Therefore, special practices, such as meditation to quiet and expand one's mental faculties; breath control, which allowed the development of one's internal and physical energy; and specific movement techniques, which gave one the ability to actually express this energy and power were used, bringing about true metamorphosis and integration of body, mind, and spirit.... This missing factor or element in Western philosophy has given way to a superficial means of self-realization: it only exists in our ego and nowhere else.

-Wayne B. Chandler, Ancient Future (Black Classic Press, 1999. p 214)

4.

Tai Chi and the African-Asian Connection

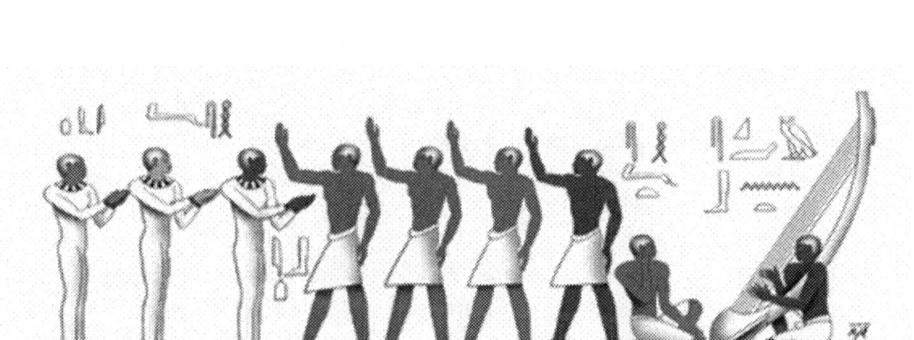

In this illustration, hand clapping and music accompany various exercises in Kemet. *Courtesy, Nijart International*

The word, *Afriasian*, used in the title of this book signifies the connection between two cultures. Throughout the history of African-Asian cultures, including and beginning with ancient Egypt, Babylonia, Mesopotamia, India, Japan and China, a strong link has existed between mind, body and spirit development, belief systems, fighting arts of warfare, and the healing arts and sciences. This phenomenon has been called by many names in these various cultures: *Ra/Ankh* (Kemet or ancient Egypt), *Nkra* (West Africa), *Ase* (Yorubaland/Nigeria), *Ntu* (southern Africa), *Prana* (India), *Ki* (Japan), and *Chi/Qi* (China).

I adhere to a self-imposed mandate that the contributions and cultural legacy of black people of the ancient and modern world attain recognition, not only by oral traditions, but also in writing. Most books, films, research articles, and various other reference materials that discuss the martial arts tend to gloss over certain African-Asiatic names, dynasty dates, and/or cultural implications or differences. I agree with others that acknowledgement of cultural contributions to the history of martial arts must extend beyond Korea, Japan, Okinawa and China. As a student of the Egyptian philosophical system of *MAAT*, I, in agreement with others, have recognized the similarity between it and the philosophy of the Tao. For many years I have also practiced *Kupigana Ngumi*, a fighting style developed based on research about Kemet. In the book, *Kupigana Ngumi: Root Symbols of the Ntchru and Ancient Kmt, Volume I*, similarities to the Asian concepts appear. For instance, certain animal symbols represent the laws of nature embodied by that animal and not worship of the animal. According to my mentors, Shaha Mfundishi Maasi and Nganga Mfundishi Tolo-Naa, the following are some examples:

> HERU—the falcon, family of the hawk and eagle, is fast and powerful and can gaze into the sun
> JHUTY—the crane is soft and gentle but has a deadly fighting style
> ENPU—the sacred black jackal symbolizing transformation
> UATCHET—the snake commands fear for it power, force and sense of feeling

This symbolism was but a method used to identify and clarify the essential function of a law of nature. Because of this and other similarities, I was curious about the existence of an African-Asian connection in Tai Chi. According to the *Kupigana Ngumi* research, weapons and fighting arts have been a legitimate and prominent part of both Indonesian and African cultures from ancient times. The researchers show that the early civilizations of India and Africa shared an intimate social, cultural and genetic link. As a long-time instructor of various martial arts within the urban community of Louisville, Kentucky, USA, I know the value of a sense of community among the youth and adults who were my students throughout the years. Many believed that the study of the martial arts was not for them—rather it was for the Chinese or Japanese or other Asians. However, whenever my classes met we took time to reframe the learning of the art within the context of our identity because the training is universal. As a black person, I continue to be encouraged to discover and uncover the possible contributions of the descendents of African societies to the discipline that has been such an integral part of my own life. Therefore, I include this section primarily as 'food for thought' and perhaps as an expanded way of looking at the martial arts—and Tai Chi specifically—for people of African descent. It is important to note that some people do not agree with these findings.

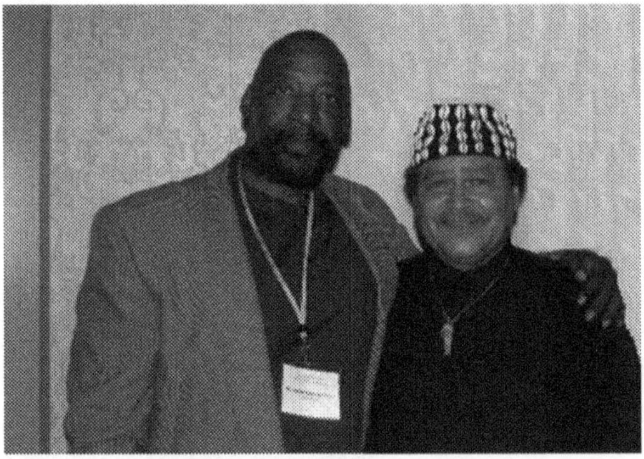

Mfundishi Serikali with Dr. Asa Hilliard at the Black Family Conference, Louisville, KY (2004)
Photo courtesy of RamImages.com

At the Fernback Museum of Natural History in Atlanta, Georgia there is a great visual display depicting the origin and dispersion of humankind around the globe. The path from Ethiopia of Eastern Africa through Mesopotamia, Arabia and Persia on through India, China and the Far East are easily visible. The archeological records and linguistic and mythological correspondences show that in the early times of antiquity, a single group who shared cultural, social and genetic relations, before a northern invasion, populated the entire area from Ethiopia to southern Eurasia to China. According to archaeological finds, the oldest hominoids in the world lived in Africa long before they appeared anywhere else. Dr. Asa G. Hilliard, III is the Fuller E. Callaway Professor of Urban Education at Georgia State University, with joint appointments in the Department of Educational Policy Studies and the Department of Educational Psychology/Special Education and Atlanta University. A teacher, psychologist, and historian, Dr. Hilliard has written more than two hundred research reports, articles and books on testing, ancient African History, teaching strategies, African culture, and child growth and development. Dr. Hilliard has consulted with many of the leading school districts, publishers, public advocacy organizations, universities, government agencies and private corporations on valid assessment, African content in curriculum, teacher training, and public policy. Several of his programs in curriculum, assessment, and valid teaching have become national models. His books include *Free Your Mind, Return to the Source: The African Origin of Civilization* (San Francisco: Urban Institute for Human Services, 1978) and *SBA: The Reawakening of The African Mind* (Gainesville, Florida: Makare Publishing, 1997). Dr. Hilliard makes several observations in his writings:

- The oldest recorded civilization to date is the Nile Valley civilization
- The oldest nation on record to date was the Nubian nation located to the south of Kemet
- "Kemet" means "land of the blacks"
- Kemet was Africa's greatest recorded classical civilization
- Only in the last one million years do we find that hominoids were on other continents one million years after the Nile Valley civilization

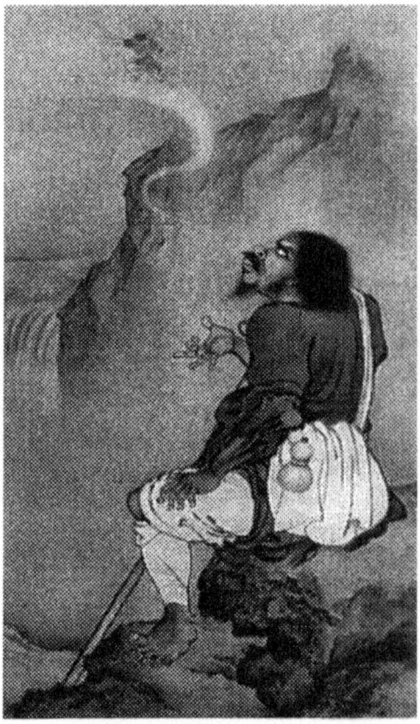

Li Tieguai, the healer

In Chinese mythology, the image of one of the Eight Immortals, Li Tieguai[4], bears the resemblance of one born of African ancestry. In addition, a great deal of research about the history and origins of the Chinese people and their philosophies comes from the work of Professor Albert Etienne Jean Baptiste Terrien de Lacouperie

[4] In Chinese Daoism one will find The Eight Chinese Immortals who are legendary beings based on historical characters. These beings, at different periods and for various reasons, each attained immortality. Each one of the immortals represents a different condition in life, i.e., poverty, wealth, aristocracy, plebeians, age, youth, masculinity and femininity. The Eight Chinese Immortals were Li Tieguai, Han Zhongli, Lan Caihe, Zhang Guolao, He Xiangu, LuDongbing, Han Xiangzi, and CaoGuojiu. Each of the immortals bear one of the attributes of the eight Daoist emblems. Stories of the Eight Immortals can be found in Chinese art forms, in folklore, drama, novels, and woodblock prints.

(1845–1894). He was an English sinologist with appointments as Professor of Indo-Chinese Philology at the University of London, and President of the Council of the Royal Asiatic Society and Philological Society. As an accomplished philologist, Professor Lacouperie authored 25 books that are read in three languages (Chinese, French and English) including *Blacks in Ancient China* (New Haven: Yale University Press, 1887. Reprint 1987.) and *Western Origin of the Early Chinese Civilization* (Osnaloruck: Otto Zeller, 1894. Reprint 1966.) Lacouperie identified a group of families known as the *Bak* who immigrated into China from a country immediately East of Babylonia. According to Lacouperie, the *Bak* are responsible for the transfer of knowledge into China. He maintains that they carried with them the sociopolitical structure, writing, philosophy, and economic fortification necessary to begin a civilization. Using various historical documents, he goes on to show that this group was culturally related to the Meso-Sumerians of West Asia, while racially and ethnically the *Bak* were descendents of the Black Akkadians and Elamites of Mesopotamia. In the early 20th century, many anthropologists, such as Professor George A. Dorsey of Chicago, believed that dark-skinned people with kinky hair originally inhabited this whole region of the world bordering the Indian Ocean.

Admittedly, Tai Chi can trace its roots back to ancient India through the Buddhist monk, Bodhidharma. His name has various spellings in three cultures. Among them, he is also known as Ta Mo [also Talmo or Da Mo or Dot Mor] in China and Daruma [also Bodai Daruma or Dharuma or Darumasan] in Japan and is credited for bringing Mahayana Buddhism to the Orient between 540 A.D. and 525 A.D. Bodhidharma was a great Indian sage who was born in the southern Indian kingdom of Pallva where he resided in Kanchi, one of its largest cities. Born between 483 A.D. and 440 A.D., the third son of a Brahman king of the Sardili clan, well educated according to his time, he was proficient in the arts, politics, sutras and warfare. He was not quite thirty when he left the princely comforts to dedicate his life to attaining enlightenment. Having become a reputable monk, he went to China to propagate the teachings of Buddha, as many of his Indian predecessors had done.

Bodhidharma was a Dravidian, a member of the black aboriginal population that dominated most of Asia during his time, the last of the twenty-eight patriarchs of India, and the first of the six patriarchs of China. As an adult Bodhidharma journeyed to China bringing with him the ancient Indian martial arts that once permeated Indian society. While there, he visited the Shaolin monks in the Hunan [Honan] Province. The resident Chinese monks were in awe of Bodhidharma's mastery of meditation. Accordingly, he redefined the Chinese approach to

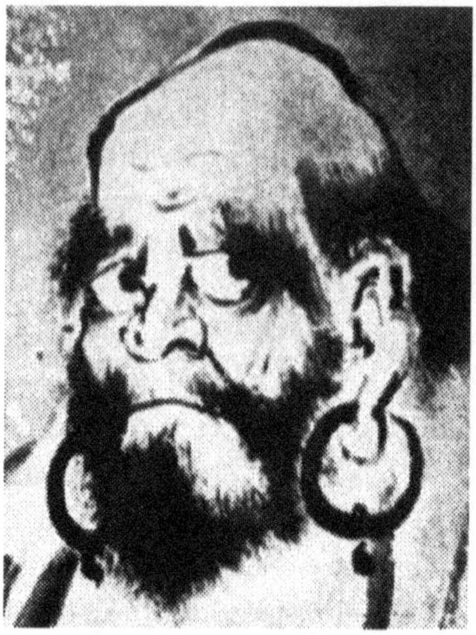

Bodhidharma/Ta Mo/Dharuma

Buddhism. His contribution, now known as Chan Buddhism in China and Zen Buddhism in Japan, required long periods of meditation rather than adherence to a particular doctrine or scripture. Bodhidarma believed in the necessity of physical discipline, which he saw lacking in the monks' daily routine. He taught them breathing techniques designed to strengthen and condition their bodies and build inner energy and endurance. He also taught the monks movement techniques to foster strength and their self-defense skills. These exercises were the forerunners of the external approach in martial arts and were based on the practice of yoga in India. Later, in China, yoga developed into what is called *Shaolin Chuan*. That is why Bodhidharma is credited with forming the groundwork for all modern kung fu, or *wu shu*, which includes Tai Chi.

This is all very interesting because of the strong evidence regarding the roots of the civilizations of India. Professor Ernest Albert Hooten (1887–1954), a Rhodes Scholar at Oxford University with a strong interest in physical anthropology, archaeology, and prehistory who later join Harvard as an anthropologist made the following statement:

> A large share of the responsibility for the great civilization of India must be assigned to Negroes, since there is unquestionably a strong Negroid strain in the Indian population.
>
> —*Up from the Ape* (New York: Macmillan Company, 1946, p. 591)

Indeed, although the cultural relations between India and China can be traced back to very early times, there is evidence that India's influence upon China is the result of Africa's influence on India. Indian historian and anthropologist Bharatiya Vidya Bhavan asserts:

> We have to begin with the Negroid or Negrito people of prehistoric India who were its first human inhabitants. Originally, they would appear to have come from Africa through Arabia and the coastlands of Iran and Baluchistan…
>
> —*The Vedic Age*, Volume I, 1962

Just as humanity's journey on the earth followed discernable patterns, so also I believe that the proliferation of knowledge traced the same footsteps. In other words, knowledge understandably comes from older, established civilizations to younger, less stable ones.

So then, the story of the development of a form similar to what is now known as Tai Chi having roots in Kemet seems highly plausible. My best effort to trace this story results in references to the research of Rev. Sterling M. Means, a historian in the 1940s. According to Means, the teaching of this form called Ku-Ta, meaning "defender of kings", to the royal bodyguards protected the Pharaohs of Kemet. Ku-Ta was a privately taught and secretly practiced form. Just as in the history of Tai Chi, Ku-Ta passed from generation to generation to the bodyguards of the rulers in Asia where it remained secret among Asian rulers for over one thousand years. Perhaps this, too, was due to the influence of African principles. According to Dr. Hilliard, "African teachers respect mastery, and seek through apprenticeship to learn from true masters." The main principle of this form was the use of the whole body as one complete unit like a coiled spring exploding into shock waves of vibrating "whip-like" energy called *fa-jing* by the Chinese. It is believed that Ku-Ta was eventually passed on to China where it was renamed Kun-Tao and continued to teach students how to move as one complete unit—body/mind/spirit—with no expression of duality as in Tai Chi, yet emphasizing the physical.

Finally, others presently continue to document the African trail through the civilizations of history. Wayne B. Chandler is an historian, photographer and the author of many books and articles. His contemporaries have given him the title of "anthrophotojournalist" because of his expert knowledge in several disciplines that he uses to approach history. His photography shows the features of faces that are undeniably of African descent on pottery, cave carvings, and other treasures of various cultures. According to historians such as Mr. Chandler and Ivan Van Sertima (author of *African Presence in Early Asia*), two of China's earliest dynasties, the Shang and the Shia [also Xia] were both heavily Black African/Black Oceanic dynasties, along with Mongol Chinese as well. They dominated China about 2800 B.C. to 1100 B.C. Researcher Clyde Winters also continues to investigate and document evidence of an African connection to many of the world's first civilizations. According to him, the analogy between the Manding and Chinese languages suggest that Manding language is a foundation of the Chinese language. Because of this, he also claims, the view that some early rulers of China came from the Kunte clan and were Manding speakers must be a consideration. Finally, Professor Runoko Rashidi is a historian, research specialist, writer, world traveler, and public lecturer focusing on the African presence globally and the African foundations of world civilizations. His passion is regarding the African presence in Asia, Australia, and the Pacific Islands. I, too, share this passion for helping to change the way the world views Africa by studying those connections that have been lost, forgotten or erased.

I hope that you now have enough information to ponder. This section has been of particular importance to me because of the pervasive impetus to remove Egypt and the "upper" Nile civilizations from association with "black" Africa. Do not allow others to rewrite history in this manner. Surely, now you have no reason to believe that Tai Chi is not for you or that the philosophy is not a part of your own ancestry. It is helpful for our bodies, minds and spirits. As the origin of all people and philosophies everywhere has a single beginning, we all can embrace Tai Chi as our own, with singleness of mind. I have permission. Whatever your cultural lineage may be—YOU have permission.

The purpose of T'ai Chi Ch'uan is to develop civil and martial accomplishment and to heal the nations.

-Master Yang Lu Chan

5

Tai Chi and Health

The grandson of Yang Lu Chan, Yang Cheng Fu, is often called the "father of modern Tai Chi" because of his role in popularizing the art during the 1930's. Allegedly, he told the story of being disillusioned with the study of Tai Chi as a young boy because it only enabled him to defend himself against one person at a time. He wanted to learn a technique that would enable him to fight many at once, by which means he could help save China from being conquered and divided up by other nations. His uncle explained to him that Tai Chi was not just a means of self-defense, but it was also a method of making people healthier and stronger. In order to save a nation, his uncle continued, he could start by making his people healthy and strong. Then there would be some hope of saving the country from foreign domination. From that time on, Yang Cheng Fu dedicated himself to learning and teaching Tai Chi with emphasis on the immense benefits to health and longevity.

After the advent of gunpowder rendered the martial art aspect of Tai Chi less potent a weapon for defense, the Yang family began to concentrate on the health aspect of the art, recognizing that a common enemy of man is disease. The Yang practitioners sought to ward off ill health with the same philosophy formerly used to ward off their human attackers. It is this link, then, this lineage of Yang style for health and longevity that has today excited the holistic medical community the world over and it is this connection with the Yang family of healers that motivates me to follow through with a commitment to enhance the lives of others through education. I am convinced that as we learn more about Tai Chi the emphasis naturally shifts to equipping the populace with knowledge to improve health because of the overwhelming pressures today to become and remain health-conscious. As an African American, I am acutely aware of the various diseases and ailments that afflict my own people so that the advice of Yang Cheng Fu's uncle is very much a part of my specific goals for the advancement of Tai Chi.

No matter what the theories of the origin of Tai Chi may be, it is an accepted fact that emphasis in Tai Chi shifted from aspects that are more combative to health and body-mind harmony during the mid-19th century. From then on, Tai Chi has primarily evolved into a health-oriented exercise that is a popular practice by people of all ages for its health benefits. Estimates are that over 100 million people through the world practice Tai Chi on a regular basis. It is a firm belief of TCM (Traditional Chinese Medicine) that good mental and physical health is closely dependent upon the proper flow of *chi* through the body. If *chi* is weak or blocked, illness can result and can only be cured by restoring the proper flow of *chi*. Tai Chi is one method for manipulating the flow of *chi* throughout the body to aid in restoring and maintaining good health. Improvement depends not on outer strength, but inner awareness as the mind directs *chi* from the *dan tian* [also dan tien or tan tien] throughout the body. This area of the body known as "the power center" is located in the center of the body approximately two and one half inches below the navel. It is the balance point within the body itself. It is the single, live meditation point during the entire series of movements. The gentle Tai Chi movements drawing power from the *dan tian* and coupled with concentration and inner awareness are, according to TCM, one of the keys to natural health and immunity to degenerative diseases.

From my perspective this is the most exciting part of this book. Despite the fact that there is very little scientific evidence confirming the special health benefits of Tai Chi, various empirical studies concerning relaxation and meditation research have placed Tai Chi in the forefront of disciplines worth pursuing in large studies. Tai Chi does not cure; Tai Chi balances the body, mind and spirit to create the environment for the body to heal itself.

Meanwhile, individuals and research trials continue to report the positive effects of Tai Chi on health and a variety of "quality of life" issues. I believe that Tai Chi is a **complete** exercise because it: 1) requires total mental concentration and clarity of mind to train the central nervous system and promote mental relaxation; 2) exercises and benefits all of the internal organs of the body, either directly or indirectly; and 3) also exercises all of the muscles, joints and ligaments of the body. Practice requires the student to apply multi-dimensional thinking. Movements

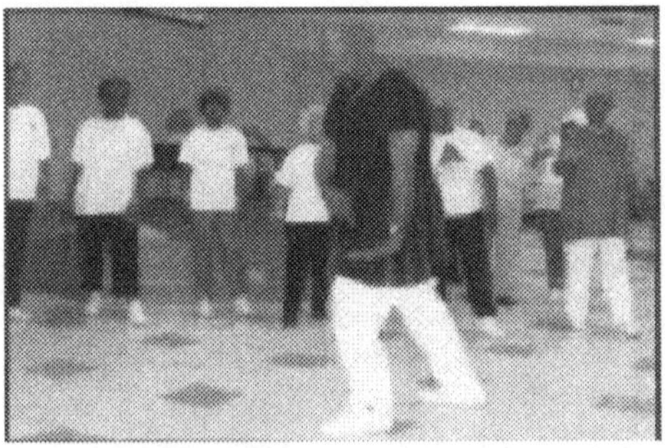

Class time in Louisville

also work both sides of the body and thus are said to work both sides of the brain. Regular practice will improve mental health, mental relaxation and the ability to concentrate. From my work with senior citizens, I watch as Tai Chi repeatedly rejuvenates participants after regular practice. Their vitality and newfound vigor becomes evident to those around them and they become the best spokespersons for the benefits of Tai Chi. Just imagine the long-term benefits for someone starting earlier in life and continuing to practice with regularity an exercise that works the body and the mind simultaneously!

Studies have shown that Tai Chi also affects physical health by improving many of the systems of the body such as the cardio-vascular, respiratory and digestive systems. It is reported to tone and strengthen the muscles gently while also improving the immune system, balance, posture, coordination, and total body awareness. Practicing triggers health and healing benefits from both the Asian paradigm of energy and the Western paradigm of physiology. The balance and flow of one's internal self healing energies is enhanced by the slow, meditative movements of Tai Chi. At the very same time the delivery of oxygen and nutrition from the blood to the tissues is improved. The lymph system's ability to eliminate metabolic by-products and transport immune cells is increased. The biochemical profile of the brain and nervous system is shifted toward recovery and healing. To attain the sense of connectedness needed to sustain balance, the student must look at and resolve or heal any obstruction blocking the way. In Tai Chi issues are resolved effectively over time because practice requires that a large amount of attention be focused toward self; initially to the body, but eventually to every level. So, Tai Chi uses a method of relaxing muscle tension, improving posture and deepening of the breathing process to positively change the stress levels of the mind and the emotions. In my research I have found claims that Tai Chi has been successfully used in cases involving mental stress, heart disease, hypertension, diabetes, arthritis, chronic pain, insomnia, asthma, lupus, fibromyalgia, AIDS, Parkinson's, Multiple Sclerosis, Sickle Cell Anemia, etc. There are also various sources documenting Tai Chi as a viable adjunct therapy to treat pain and various psychosomatic diseases. In this chapter I want to point out some of the findings from research along with the claims from those who have benefited from the practice of Tai Chi in the hopes that as you read you will consider how practicing Tai Chi can be a beneficial addition to your health regimen.

As stated before, there have been numerous reports of improved conditions and even some cures attributed to Tai Chi. Much of the research has been carried out in China but some has also been undertaken in other parts of the world as the popularity of Tai Chi increased. For example, the National Institute on Aging studied frailty and injuries in elderly patients:

> Tai Chi, a martial arts form that enhances balance and body awareness through slow, graceful, and precise body movements, can significantly cut the risk of falls among older people and may be beneficial in maintaining gains made by people age 70 and older who undergo other types of balance and strength training. The news comes in two reports appearing in the May 1996 issue of the Journal of the American Geriatrics Society. In the first study, Steven L. Wolf, Ph.D., and colleagues at the Emory University School of Medicine, Atlanta, Ga., found that older people taking part in a 15-week Tai Chi program reduced their risk of falling by 47.5 percent. A second study, by Leslie Wolfson, M.D., and colleagues at the University of Connecticut Health Center, Farmington, found that several interventions to improve balance and strength among older people were effective. These improvements, particularly in strength, were preserved over a 6-month period while participants did Tai Chi exercises.
>
> —National Institute of Health Press Release, May/1996

More information regarding the first study, *Tai Chi for the Prevention of Falls in the Elderly*, was reported in Integrative Medicine, Vol. 1, No. 4, pp. 167-169, 1998. The setting was the Atlanta Frailty and Injuries: Cooperative Studies of Intervention Techniques (FICSIT) site, a community dwelling for ambulatory elderly persons over the age of 70 years. With the stated objective being "to evaluate whether Tai Chi and computerized balance training in the community dwelling elderly reduce frailty and/or the occurrence of falls", the study concluded that "twice weekly Tai Chi classes resulted in a significant impact on biomedical and psychosocial indicators of frailty. ***More importantly, this minimal intervention*** can reduce the risk of falls by 47.5% in the elderly population." [Emphasis mine] The great benefit of Tai Chi here is that it focuses on the correct physiological use of the body or proper body mechanics and alignment making it ideal for those having physical concerns (like falling) or disabilities.

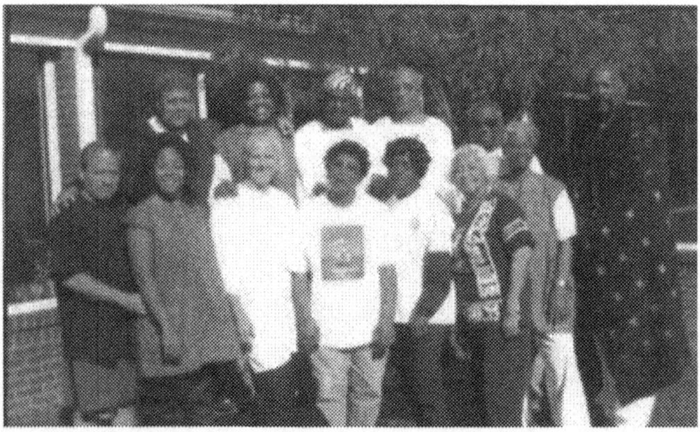

Mfundishi Serikali and members of the Oak and Acorn Tai Chi Class (Louisville, KY)

As I continue to hold classes for senior citizens, I never cease to be amazed at the positive results that seniors derive from Tai Chi practice. For a number of reasons I believe that Tai Chi is one of the best possible exercise programs for senior citizens. I attribute this in part to the fact that Tai Chi places a great emphasis on balance, both physical and mental. Since it is very common for people to lose their sense of balance and become more susceptible to falls and subsequent injuries as they age, Tai Chi is the perfect, low-impact exercise. It has been documented that the fear of falling is one of the greatest concerns of senior citizens. In Tai Chi practice, the principles of balance (including ankle, knee and hip joint involvement), lower body awareness, and posture are key components. When a relaxed, erect upper body is correctly positioned over a relaxed lower body structure, then the ability to remain balanced within movement becomes a powerful therapeutic tool utilizing gravity and skill. This leads to a better awareness of body movement and a growing confidence that permits a person of any age to live a fuller and more productive life. It is particularly good to see senior citizens move with assurance as they face the challenges of learning new skills while strengthening their legs and conditioning the tendons and ligaments.

Other major benefits, not only for seniors, are the emphasis on gentleness and relaxation and the challenge to improve flexibility and elasticity. The constant weight shifting trains balance while increasing the range of motion of the ankles, knees, and hips making them more resilient and less prone to injury. In another sense of the word, tension and stress are also expressions of imbalance. Therefore, the cultivation of improved balance as a mind/body experience can only have a reducing effect on tension and stress. The topic is also the subject of a clinical trial: "Complementary/Alternative Medicine for Abnormality in the Vestibular (Balance) System" conducted by the National Center for Complementary and Alternative Medicine (NCCAM) at Massachusetts General Hospital Biomotion

Laboratory, Boston, Massachusetts. At the time of this writing participants were still being recruited to "determine the relative merits of vestibular rehabilitation and Tai Chi for patients with inner ear (vestibular) disorders."

It is said that physical strength peaks in the mid-twenties, declines to age 50, and steeply declines thereafter. Studies claim to show a loss of one-third of lower extremity strength by age 70. In advanced age, few people are able to stand on one leg for more than a few seconds. Premature decline does not need to be a foregone conclusion for the elderly. Leg strength increases with practice of Tai Chi as the sinking of the weight, over time, tells the legs to add muscle and bone mass. Tai Chi is for anyone who wants to move with greater strength, grace, and ease as they age. Consumer Reports on Health, November 1998, page 8, cited one study published in *Medicine & Science in Sports & Exercise.* This study evaluated volunteers age 58 to 70, who practiced Tai Chi an average of five days a week. The results showed a 15 to 20 percent improvement in aerobic capacity and knee strength after one year. In a second study, presented at a meeting of the American Heart Association, researchers at Johns Hopkins School of Medicine found that older volunteers (average age: 67) with elevated blood pressure who did Tai Chi for 12 weeks lowered their systolic blood pressure by 7 mm Hg—nearly as much as those who did a moderately intense aerobic-exercise program of walking and low-impact aerobics. Both groups did their respective exercise for 30 minutes, four times a week.

I did not cite any of many studies involving the effects of stress because there are so many of them. What condition isn't adversely affected by stress? One of the greatest contributory factors of health problems in modern America has been the staggering effect of stress, not only on the physical, but also on the mental and emotional states of today's busy corporate types. Most doctors agree that it is not the stress itself that is the real villain, but how the individual views the stress and deals with it that is important. There is already a plethora of articles, books, exercises and workshops designed just to educate the public on how to deal with the subject in our daily lives. It has been said that more than 50% of illnesses treated by modern doctors can be attributed to psychosomatic disorders or, directly or indirectly, to mental stress. We well know that mental stress can cause physical illnesses such as high blood pressure. Stress has been proven to cause increased blood cholesterol levels and even some forms of cancer. Thus mental stress has a very clear and direct relationship to total body health, causing not only mental but also physical illness. With all the many ways of relieving stress today, why should anyone take time for Tai Chi?

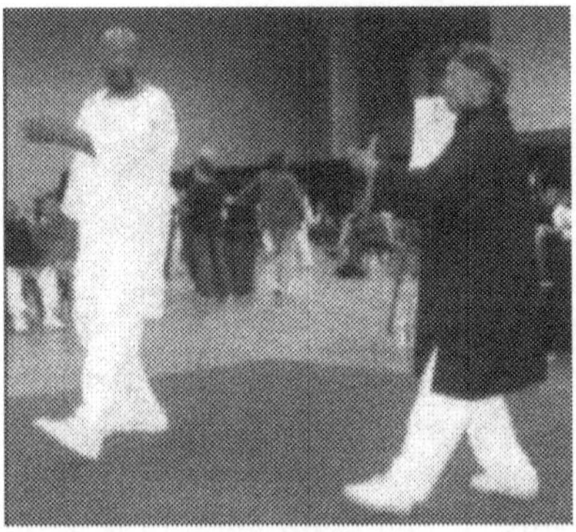

Preparing for competition

In TCM, stress and tension are imbalances blocking the flow of *chi* through the body. Tai Chi principles show immense promise for helping psychotherapy generate emotional and spiritual growth in addition to solving problems. The synthesis of Tai Chi and psychology gives birth to a new kind of psychotherapy wherein emotional problems are addressed on an energy level and healing occurs in the client's energy system itself. External changes in behavior, thought and feeling are generated by freeing the client's *chi*. Tai Chi principles empower psychotherapy to generate holistic growth. By far, the most sought after benefits of practicing Tai Chi are relaxation of mind and body to combat the stresses of daily life. This makes Tai Chi so practical for the workplace and corporate wellness programs. Just as massage therapy has made its way into the corporate arena, so is Tai Chi advancing. It takes a relatively short amount of time to do and provides benefits that any employer would appreciate. Often employees report that they are able to not only meet the pressures and challenges at work with more equilibrium but also are able to focus on work for longer periods of time. A complete article on the subject was written by Harriet Lynn of Communications Health/Network, Inc. of Baltimore, Maryland in which she states:

> Ironically, the timeless holistic fitness system of Taijiquan meets the modern criteria for keeping all employees health in mind, body, and spirit. At the same time Taijiquan, which some translate as "Supreme Ultimate", complies to the needs of the bottom line of a company. Taijiquan can be inexpensively implemented while keeping employee productivity levels high.

Tai Chi can be a way to take control and place limits on the way your body deals with the pressures of life because there is a direct physiological connection between relaxing the mind and relaxing the body. The *Harvard Health Letter* (21:11, 1996) reported that researchers at La Trobe University in Australia found that Tai Chi was as effective as meditation and brisk walking in reducing the levels of some stress hormones in men and women both during and after practice. Once a basic Tai Chi form is learned, the practice of it produces a meditation state and, thus, greater production of anti-stress hormones (ACTH). Regular practice has an enduring benefit to both the physical and psychological tolerance of stress through the lowering of blood lactate levels and the increase in endorphin production. The sense of calmness is no accident! The mind is clear and alert in order to direct and coordinate the movement of all parts of the body. This exercises the central nervous system and improves mental relaxation. Tai Chi promotes a sense of overall well-being and "alert relaxation." It creates a tranquil state of mind through concentration on the movements. This is the body's restraint on the flight or fight syndrome and is of vital importance in lessoning the effects of negative stress. In practicing Tai Chi the principle requirement is for the mind to be completely cleared of extraneous thought so that the mind can completely focus on the execution of the required movements. When good Tai Chi is practiced, the muscles are gently stretched out and fully relaxed as is only possible with a relaxed mind. This stretching strengthens both the muscles and the bones, making the muscles and stronger more supple. To accomplish this, it is necessary to train the mind to reach a mental state similar to that of meditation.

My research also located a reference to a 1980 a study conducted targeting African Americans in the United States who deal with the genetic stressor of the negative sociopolitical, cultural, and religious attitudes associated with skin color. Titled "A Theoretical Model of Psychosomatic Illness in Blacks and An Innovative Treatment Strategy" it was reported in the Journal of Black Psychology by C. Mack and is of special interest to me as a black male. The participants, males with pre-program conditions of headaches, restlessness, hypertension, constipation, and ulcerated stomachs, were part of a 24-week program of Tai Chi instruction. Their post-program surveys noted a significant difference in their awareness of and reaction to stressful events along with other findings. Mack attributed the results to the relaxation response of Tai Chi. He further stated that Tai Chi relieved somatic stress more quickly than deep meditation and indeed provided African Americans with an alternative method to deal with either situational or genetic stress.

Another experiment measured brain wave activity (EEG) for two groups of people. One group consisted of regular practitioners of Tai Chi while the other group was a control group not practicing Tai Chi. A larger number of alpha waves were recorded for the group of Tai Chi practitioners than for the control group. This is important because there is a lot of basic knowledge about what alpha waves are and what makes them appear and disappear in our brains. Alpha waves do appear and disappear—they are not always present. For example, in deep sleep there are no alpha waves, and if someone is very highly aroused as in fear or anger, again there are virtually no alpha waves. So, the greater production of alpha waves in this experiment signified a greater state of mental clarity, calmness, and concentration. Some have conjectured that the positive effects of Tai Chi may be solely due to the fact that it is known that stress reduction occurs as we perform activities we find pleasurable and/or satisfying that distract us from problems and anxiety. I say that even if this proves to be true, it is a good thing to find an alternative to the "no pain—no gain" route for exercise and deep meditation for the mind.

Various studies have shown that regular practice of Tai Chi improves heart function by exercising the heart in a gentle, yet gradual and well-controlled way, in a manner similar to swimming. Dr. Wen Zee[5], a retired cardiologist in Shanghai, believes that Tai Chi is "an incomparable exercise because it never accelerates the heart rate." He believes that exercises such as running and jogging can injure the heart and a person can easily meet the standards set by the American Heart Association by practicing Tai Chi three times a day. Dr. John Painter[6], a Fort Worth, Texas based teacher of internal Chinese martial arts, claims that "when the movements of Tai Chi are performed quickly or in a lower formed stance, they have the same beneficial effect on the cardiovascular system as jogging or high-impact aerobics, but without the stress and strain." According to HealthWorld Online, some have cited studies showing that twenty minutes of Tai Chi gives participants 80% of the same cardiovascular benefit as aerobics.

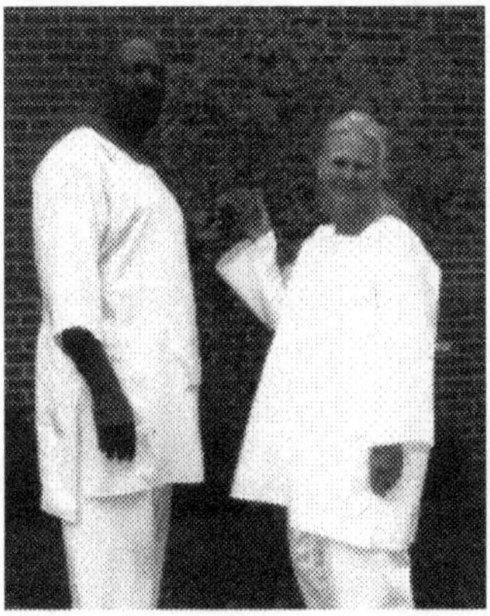

Mfundishi and student

While the argument for or against Tai Chi alone as a tool for achieving aerobic fitness continues, there is no argument that exercising the cardiovascular system in Tai Chi is gentle yet continuous and can be tailored to suit different levels of health. Another means by which the heart benefits from the practice of Tai Chi is through the abdominal breathing techniques. In Tai Chi, deep breathing is never imposed on the student; it is developed step

[5] Dr. Wen Zee, formerly of Shanghai, China, came to the United States in 1993. From 1994 to 1997, he served as a visiting scientist at the University of Arizona, College of Medicine. He currently teaches Chinese herbal medicine and Tai Chi Chuan classes in Tucson, Arizona.

[6] For more information on Dr. John P. Painter, visit www.ninedragonbaguazhang.com/drp.htm

by step. The student gradually learns to coordinate his breathing with the movements. The deep breathing promoted by the slow practice of Tai Chi causes the diaphragm to expand outwards and downwards and contract inwards and upwards. This deep breathing causes increasing and decreasing pressure inside the abdominal cavity which, in turn, causes the same effect inside the thoracic cavity giving the heart a gentle massage. The movement of the diaphragm also gently massages the liver and intestines. Changes of pressure inside the thoracic cavity also improve the ability of the heart and lungs to contract and expand, aiding in blood circulation and air exchange within the lungs. In improving blood circulation, more oxygen also expands the blood vessels which serve the heart and intestines helping to prevent thrombosis among other ailments.

Another factor which can lead to improved functioning of the cardiovascular system is that when the muscles of the body are stretched, especial when executing spiral movements, this has an effect similar to that of twisting a sponge—efficiently emptying the blood and lymphatic fluid from all parts of the body including the extremities. The subsequent returning movement has an effect like untwisting a sponge—the body is able to pull in a greater amount of blood and nutrients than normal. Again, this improves the circulation of blood throughout the body and allows oxygen to reach all parts of the body more efficiently.

There are other factors affecting the heart, such as cholesterol and triglyceride levels, that can be decreased through the practice of Tai Chi. Stimulation of the central nervous system increases the well-being of all of the organs of the body. Holding the spine in correct alignment and turning and moving the waist helps the student to stimulate the parasympathetic nervous system. This causes a decrease in heart rate and dilation of the blood vessels resulting in improvement in the circulation. All of the Tai Chi movements enhance the circulation of blood throughout the body. In Traditional Chinese Medicine (TCM) health is evaluated based on the quality and amount of blood circulation; good circulation is good health.

Tai Chi may be the best exercise to add to a routine aimed at heart conditions such as high blood pressure. Blood pressure reductions in some Tai Chi participants have been found to be only slightly less than those from a moderate-intensity aerobic exercise such as walking. Another article from HealthWorld Online cites a report from The British Medical Association's Postgraduate Medical Journal stating that Tai Chi can help heart attack victims recover faster as the slow movements and controlled breathing actually lowered blood pressure and slowed some heart rates. While one group participated in Tai Chi, another group participated in aerobic exercises. According to that article, the report showed that while both forms of exercise reduced blood pressure, only Tai Chi showed a significant reduction. In general, however, Tai Chi should be practiced along with regular, moderate aerobic exercise for good care of the cardiovascular system to achieve maximum heart-healthy benefits.

The regulated abdominal breathing required in Tai Chi is performed in conjunction with body movements and is deep, slow and rhythmic in nature. This type of deep breathing utilizes the abdominal diaphragmatic muscles and is also very beneficial for the lungs. It opens up the full space of the lungs and promotes better oxygenation of the body tissues. I have already mentioned how the creation of alternating negative and positive pressures within the thoracic and abdominal cavities improves perfusion on the internal organs. Correct coordination of body movement with breathing is very important. Inhaling should occur when a movement is performed that opens up the body, such as when both of the upper limbs stretch out. The movement involved in opening up stretches out the muscles of the chest wall, which control inspiration, as well as lowering the diaphragmatic muscles. The combination of all of these movements of the muscles fully extends the respiratory capacity. When performing a closing up movement, the reverse is also true, with all the air being fully exhaled from the lungs. In Tai Chi the lungs are stimulated directly by the constant expanding and contracting movement of the upper limbs. A quote from Traditional Chinese Fitness Exercises by China Sports Magazine and New World Press indicated that the results of a respiratory function test showed that Tai Chi practitioners enjoy greater vital lung capacity, greater lung tissue elasticity and a lower rate of calcification of the rib cartilage, as well as easier breathing patterns than those of a control group not practicing Tai Chi. Recovery time from illness is often quicker for a healthy and strong respiratory system where more oxygen is delivered to the muscles and organs. A good supply of oxygen to the organs is essential for health and the efficient burning of calories. The author of *The Catabolic Diet* even ran the following ad promoting the benefits of improved oxygenation of the body:

> Did you know that you can turn up your body's metabolism even more by simply breathing better? That's right…Most people are shallow breathers. This lowers your immune system and fails to rid your body of all the nasty toxins you consume every day. We'll teach you how to supply so much more oxygen to your system that you start ridding yourself of these toxins and skyrocket your metabolism thereby turning your body into a **FAT BURNING MACHINE**!

Tai Chi also improves the digestive system. First of all, the elimination of mental stress alone aids better digestion and the general repair and maintenance of the body. Secondly, the flow of blood to the intestines and stomach is increased through the alternating pressure inside the abdomen resulting from abdominal breathing and the twisting and turning motions of the upper body. With improved blood circulation, the function of the digestive system naturally improves also. Again, the abdominal organs receive a gentle massage from the alternating pressure cause by diaphragmatic breathing. Another finding is that the level of blood cholesterol and other blood fats (triglycerides) in the body can be significantly lowered by practicing Tai Chi for as little as six months. Tai Chi is particularly suitable for people with poorly functioning digestive systems, those suffering from IBS (irritable bowel syndrome), and for those who are overweight because the digestive system begins to function optimally and the body utilizes a greater proportion of its caloric intake.

The following excerpt concerning weight loss comes from Dr. Majid Ali, President and Professor of Medicine, Capital University of Integrative Medicine:

> The essential nature of obesity is down-regulation of fat-burning enzymes. The real issue is how to up-regulate these enzymes and not merely burn calories. The notion of burning calories to lose unwanted pounds of fat is pervasive in the United States. Hardly a week goes by that I do not hear someone outline his ambitious plans for exercise to burn out his excessive weight. With rare exceptions, all he gets is sore muscles, pulled tendons and bruised spirits. Exercise that causes sweating and heavy breathing and gives us tired muscles is sugar-burning exercise. I call such exercise "cortical exercise." Cortical exercise is of very limited value for up-regulation of fat-burning enzymes. Up-regulation of fat-burning enzymes requires slow, sustained exercise. I call such exercise "limbic exercise." For reversing catabolic maladaptation, an overweight person needs to know the critical difference between these two types of exercise. I discuss this subject at length in the companion volume *The Ghoraa and Limbic Exercise*. The health professional advising the obese person so often fails to see the critical difference between sugar-burning cortical and fat-burning limbic exercises. It is only when the catabolic illusion is dissipated with knowledge and insight that the obese person has any real chance of correcting his catabolic maladaptation for good…Learn how slow, sustained exercise can be combined with "limbic language" to achieve higher levels of health and spiritual awareness.

In a compendium of medical literature author Dr. Janice Weiss states (regarding Dr. Ali's method):

> He definitely does not agree with the "mind over matter" attempt at healing, but rather what he calls "energy-over-mind strategy" that "gives far superior clinical results." Because "oxidant injury disrupts patterns of electromagnetic energy in muscles" he proposes using "long-term training in slow, sustained breathing patterns with prolonged unforced expiration." He refers to this as limbic breathing, and incorporates it into exercise that he insists be easy, slow, non-goal oriented, without measurements and equipment—free and easy, either walking, swimming, bicycling, running in place, protected from weather, at least initially, but always extending the slowing of breathing—inhaling, holding, exhaling. This leads to the more meditative state—the limbic non-thinking state where healing can take place. As one attains this, spirituality becomes a part of the body-mind-spiritual healing process, with freedom from desire to control, freedom from anger, and freedom from fear.

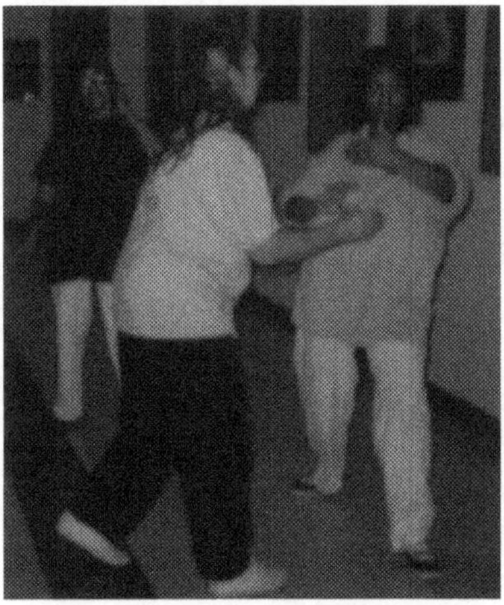

Class practice session

Science has long established that lack of physical exercise leads to a thinning and weakening of the bones (osteoporosis) and causes susceptibility to fractures. People with a deficiency of calcium combined with a lack of exercise are prone to have problems involving muscular and ligament injuries. The Traditional Chinese Fitness Exercises indicated that only 25.8% of a group of elderly Tai Chi practitioners studied suffered from spinal column deformities compared with 47.2% of a control group chosen to represent the normal population and of the same age. X-ray examination of their spines also showed senile osteoporosis in only 36.6% of the Tai Chi group as compared to 63.8% of the control group. Since regular exercise increases the density of the bones, Tai Chi is effective because as a weight-bearing exercise it increases muscle load slowly, without stress, and gradually increases the strength of the bones thereby preventing brittle bones.

In my work with seniors, I have seen improvement and reversal time and time again. When practicing Tai Chi correct and upright posture is essential. Good posture decreases the stress on the joints and the bones and allows them to work more efficiently and last longer. On the other hand, poor posture causes more stress on the joints and the bones while also affecting the internal organs. Back problems are a good example of how doing simple things poorly can lead to major trouble. Poor posture is the number one culprit in most back problems. Bending, leaning, and twisting the trunk places a great deal of stress on the lower back muscles and vertebra as they take control of the work meant for the leg muscles. Because Tai Chi trains the student to learn to move the trunk as a whole, it eliminates much of the cause of lower back pain and distress. In Tai Chi the waist is the driving part for practically every movement so that the region around the lumbar vertebrae is constantly in motion. This causes blood circulation to improve as more nutrients and oxygen are able to reach the muscles improving their nutritional state. Relaxation of upper limbs and shoulders increase circulation to the brain. The rhythmic stretching and relaxing of the muscles in Tai Chi causes them to be more supple and stronger, preventing injury or even repairing it. When performed in a slow and relaxed manner, Tai Chi offers a balanced drill for the body's muscles and joints without any buildup of lactic acid in the muscles. This drill involves the execution of complex maneuvers in conjunction with deep regulated breathing and the contraction and expansion of the diaphragm. These are the elements necessary for a high degree of joint flexibility and strength. If a joint condition such as arthritis or rheumatism is present, practice of Tai Chi can be a preventative and curative therapy.

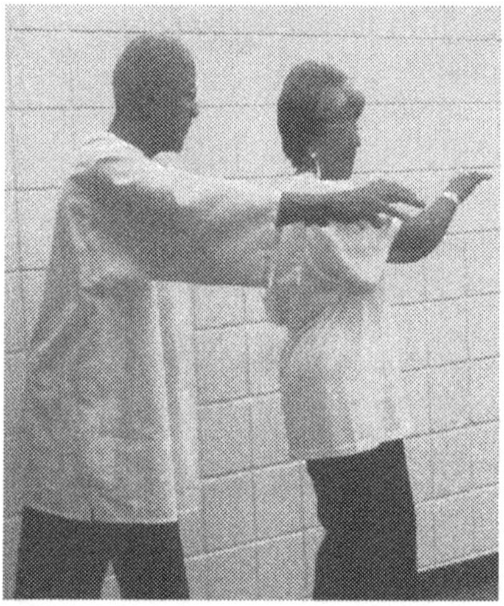

Seniors practice during class

There are reported benefits of Tai Chi for other systems in the body as well. A 2001 study reported in the Annals of Behavioral Medicine supported the effectiveness of Tai Chi in combating various other ailments. The immune system is the system of the body, which helps to fight invading disease and cleans up abnormal cells and lymph fluid is the internal cleansing agent of the body. An efficient lymphatic system subsequently helps the body to rid itself of toxins and keeps up its resistance to illness. In 1989 in Dallas, Texas, a research team undertook one of the world's largest studies on exercise and health. The findings showed that moderate exercise would improve many aspects of health, including the immunological system. Tai Chi is an entirely suitable form of exercise, such as walking or swimming, to achieve improved immunological activity. While stimulating the organs of the chest, throat and abdomen, Tai Chi also stimulates the vital glands located in these areas that are responsible for the health of the hormonal system. Since the hormonal system controls everything from sleep to reproduction, and metabolism to disease resistance, other benefits shown by this study, such as improved metabolism and regenerative capacity, also are the results of practicing Tai Chi daily. The movements of the lower abdomen and groin have a beneficial effect on blood supply to the reproductive organs. The practice of the graceful movements of Tai Chi can also lead to changes in our disposition, making us more even-tempered and slow to anger. One study involving the effects of Tai Chi on mood found that mood improved significantly during Tai Chi and remained positive one hour after practice.

The discovery that Tai Chi benefits so many different parts of the body at the same time does not diminish the level of benefit received by those individual parts. On the contrary, the benefit obtained by one system will actually enhance the benefits obtained by another. For instance, if we compare the benefit to mental relaxation obtained by practicing Tai Chi for one hour to that obtained from lying down and relaxing mentally, the former is considerably more effective because the relaxation of the muscles enhances mental relaxation, as does the abdominal breathing and the mental concentration required to perform the movements correctly. In fact, Tai Chi is so well designed that one benefit will always amplify another. The benefits compound to improve the overall health of the body in a relatively short amount of time.

Several studies and testimonials have shown positive benefits for those afflicted with certain ailments. In January of 1997 a Lupus patient, Jo Lu Roberts Johnson of Concord, NH, authored a testimonial concerning the health benefits of her regimen of Tai Chi and Qigong. She says that after her diagnosis with System Lupus Erythematosus in 1984, she had several bouts with the disease that required hospitalization for as long as eight months. Ms. Johnson further states that since beginning Tai Chi in 1995 under the guidance of her teacher she is happy to report that she has "experienced an unbroken period of good health and stronger energy with no lupus flare-ups since that time." In addition, Mary Lou Galantino, PHD, PD, wrote an article entitled, "What you should know about HIV and Tai Chi" after conducting a study in 1997. Dr. Galantino concluded that HIV patients with neuropathy or CNS opportunistic infections such as toxoplasmosis or CNF lymphoma could especially benefit from Tai Chi because these diseases bring on physical imbalance problems. She went on to further state that she would recommend the regimen even for people with HIV who are asymptomatic. In a current Tai Chi clinical trial titled, "Alternative Stress Management Approaches in HIV Disease", National Center for Complementary and Alternative Medicine (NCCAM) researchers at Virginia Commonwealth University, Richmond, Virginia are investigating whether or not people living with HIV can experience stress reduction because of practicing Tai Chi. The overall purpose of the proposed study is to determine whether three short-term stress management interventions along with booster strategies will improve and sustain improvements in the domains of psychosocial functioning, quality of life, and somatic health among persons with varying stages of HIV disease.

Similarly, Tai Chi has shown promising results for those suffering from diabetes and arthritis. *Tai Chi for Health* is a modified Sun Style Tai Chi form developed by Dr. Paul Lam to emphasize the health benefits, rather than the martial arts benefits, of Tai Chi. Dr. Lam, a family physician in Sydney, Australia, is a world leader in the field of Tai Chi for health improvement. He has produced Tai Chi programs, instructional videos, and written books that have helped many people improve their health, lifestyle and level of Tai Chi. *Tai Chi for Arthritis*, created in 1997, is a special program by Dr. Lam and a team of Tai Chi experts and eminent Rheumatologists for people with arthritis. Many Arthritis Foundations worldwide support this program. In the Winter/2000 edition of "Arthritis Today", The Arthritis Foundation of Australia clearly presented the benefits of Tai Chi for people with arthritis. Here in the United States, the Arthritis Foundation formally endorsed Tai Chi as a way to relieve the pain associated with the joint disease.

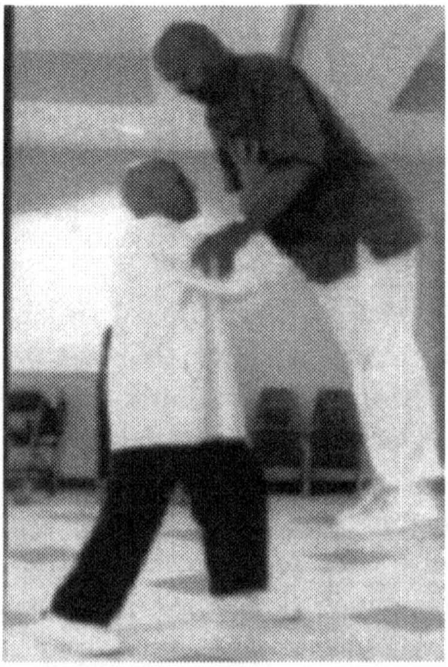

Class demo on strength training

In 2001, Dr Lam and his colleagues created the *Tai Chi for Diabetes* program which is supported by Diabetes Australia. Dr. Lam's video presents a number of different workouts specifically designed for the diabetic. Then, there is Tai Chi practitioner Bill Standen who was diagnosed with Insulin Dependent Diabetes Mellitus over fourteen years ago. In his published report on the successful treatment of his condition, he describes what happened as he practiced Tai Chi regularly. After beginning his Tai Chi practice, Bill says that he experienced a significant reduction in the amount of insulin required to control his disease. He further states that this lowered dosage was maintained with Tai Chi as the only exercise program used.

As I write this, it occurs to me that some may think that every ailment known to man will require a particular set of movements in order for Tai Chi to be effective. This is far from the truth! In actuality, while clinical trials and research do lead the way in determining the overall use of any non-traditional health program in western medicine, each of these seemingly "tailored" approaches simply reflects the particular discipline of the researcher using clients with whom there is already some familiarity. However, by looking at all of the outcomes as a whole, I maintain my conviction that Tai Chi, in any style, will benefit those who practice it and the strengthened *chi* will seek out to whatever weakness, illness or disease the body may have.

In summary, Tai Chi is a gentle from of exercise that is suitable for the entire physiological system of the human body. It is especially beneficial since it combines physical exercise with mental exercise while causing minimal injury problems. These observations have always been a part of Tradition Chinese Medicine, but how does TCM work? The basis of all TCM is the flow of internal energy throughout the body. The concept of *chi* is firmly embedded in Chinese culture and medicine. *Chi* is defined as a form of life energy which circulates all over the body in all living people. It flows from the *dan tian* along the meridians to all parts of the body. It originates as a combination of air from the lungs, the essence from the kidneys and the essence from food and drink via the digestive system. *Chi* not only maintains life and health, it governs almost all activity in the body including:

- Growth, metabolism, regeneration and repair of the body
- Regulating body temperature and keeping the organs active
- Guarding against invasion of the body by disease
- Enhancing and regulating the circulation of blood and body fluids throughout the body
- Transporting nutrients and oxygen to the whole body

A person with strong *chi* is both healthier and stronger than a person with weak *chi* and any disturbance of the flow of *chi*, or weakening of *chi*, will result in illness. *Chi* is not a tangible substance and its existence has not been detected by modern (western) scientific methods. Most Tai Chi practitioners will testify that they can feel the *chi* flowing and can, to varying degrees, direct the flow. Control of *chi* can be of great benefit in improving health. Not only does a stronger and free-flowing *chi* allow the body to function better, but it can also be directed to cure illness in a particular part of the body. For many years Traditional Chinese Medicine (TCM) doctors have recommended Tai Chi as a form of therapy. Today there are special Tai Chi units attached to many of the hospitals in China to teach patients how to use Tai Chi to improve their health. Tai Chi was created with the basic intention of strengthening internal *chi*. With a stronger *chi* and with the ability to direct it at will, the practitioner can concentrate *chi* at one point of his or her body, making this point stronger and less susceptible to injury. It is achieved by following the basic principles of Tai Chi, which allow *chi* to sink to the *dan tian* while keeping the body erect, the head straight, and relaxing and sinking the shoulder and elbow joints (rooting or grounding). The added bonus to the practitioner of Tai Chi of knowing the martial art application of the movements is that it helps to better understand how to direct the flow of internal force within it.

The dedicated practice of Tai Chi, which can greatly improve both the physical and spiritual aspects of life, can be described as the jewel of the entire holistic health care system of China—a system cloaked in secrecy for centuries. Now, after hundreds of years, the incredible benefits of the internal arts (acupuncture, reflexology, kinesiology, meridian and pressure point massage, along with a store of an entire world of herbal medicine) have finally found their universal hold. Today in medical libraries the world over there is probably as much demand for the *Yellow Emperor's Journal* as there is for the *Physician's Desk Reference*. The term *holistic* has become much more than a trendy buzzword. Holistic means that the approach to health is concerned with the entire individual. Holistic medicine does not treat the body as if it was isolated from the mind and the emotions. The world's medical community has come to realize that the various components that make up a person all interact, and when one part is adversely affected, all parts are affected. Tai Chi demonstrates this holistic approach to health in a simple and direct way.

Elson M. Haas, MD has been in medical practice for over 25 years and was instrumental in the development of the field that he has termed Integrated Medicine. He views illness as a means to change. Because a willingness to change is an integral part of Integrated Medicine, Tai Chi also merits a place among those who have adopted the use of this multidisciplinary approach to health care. There is a difference between being "not ill" and being "well" when describing our health. Choose to be healthy by doing those things that contribute to wellness. Indeed, most of us are willing to change, not because we have seen the light, but because we have felt the heat!

Although approximately 80% of the studies and experiments evaluate specific problems in the elderly or those with health problems, I want to reiterate the fact that Tai Chi is for **everyone**! The work of studies such as those mentioned in this chapter only serve to prove that if Tai Chi can affect these groups so positively, just imagine what beginning a life-long practice of Tai Chi will do for young, healthy individuals. When asked by a student "What is the most important reason to study Tai Chi Chuan?", Master Cheng Man Ching replied, "The most important reason is that when you finally reach the place where you understand what life is about, you'll have the health to enjoy it." Remember that our health is our only real material wealth! Often, however, it is only realized when it is too late.

Photo Gallery

In my earlier days of karate, I had the privilege of bestowing an honorary black belt on hometown native Muhammad Ali. Although I have since met many persons of importance, I still hold Muhammad Ali in highest esteem.

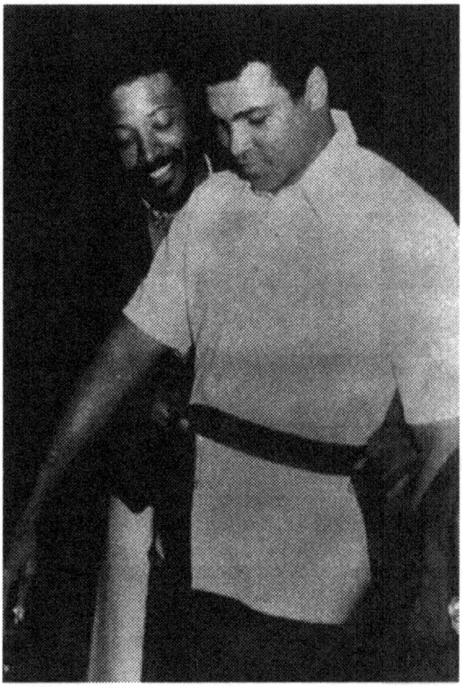

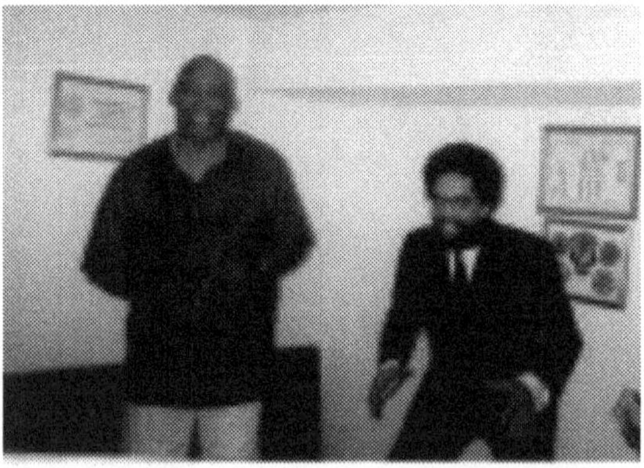

More recently, I had a chance to spend some time with Professor Cornel West. It is time that I will always treasure.

Photo Gallery

Despite the busy schedule, I had the opportunity to practice a few Tai Chi movements with Professor West.

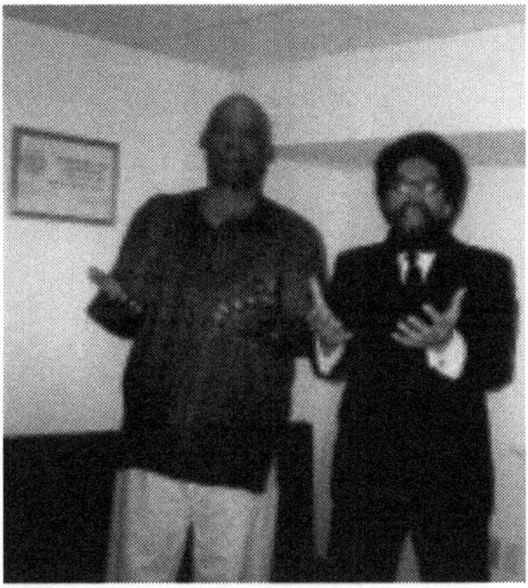

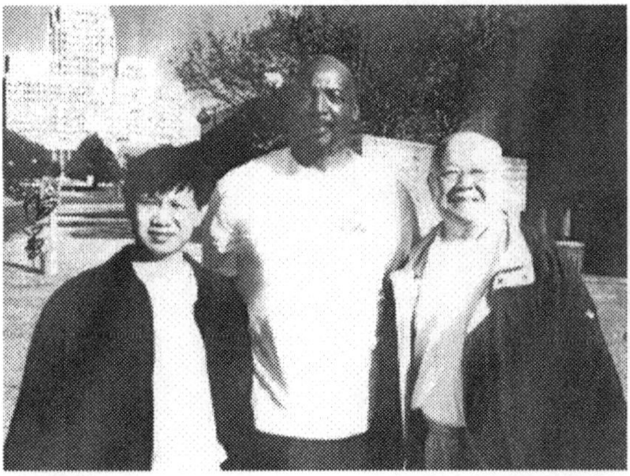

In July of 2002, I attended a Tai Chi workshop in Buffalo, New York. This workshop was special because 6th generation Yang Family descendent Master Yang Jun (left) and 4th generation Yang Family descendent Grandmaster Yang Zhen Dou (right) were very personable and complementary of my skills as they led the workshops.

Photo Gallery

Grandmaster Yang Zhen Dou found time for extra conversation and more pictures.

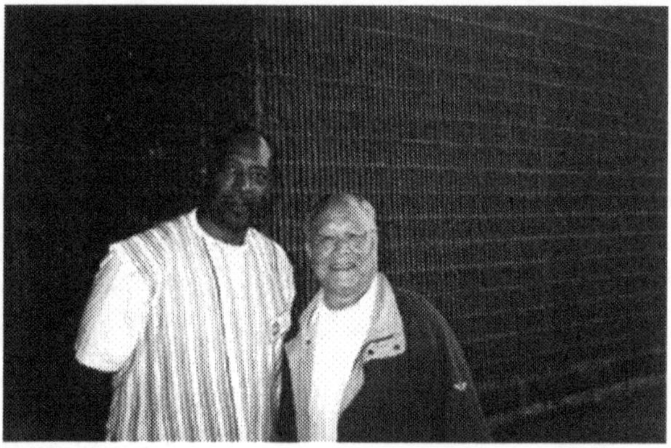

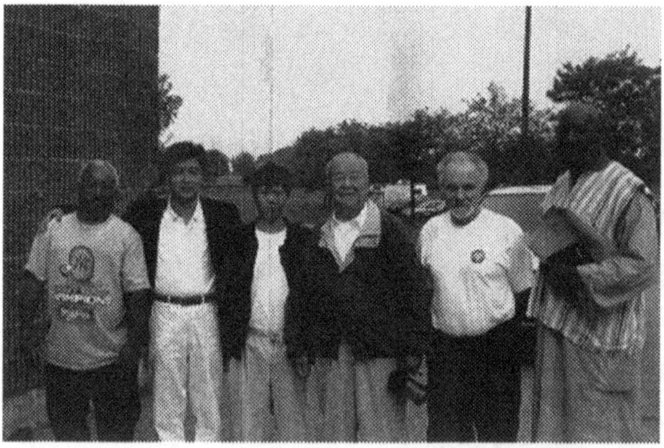

Group photo with the Yang Family descendents and several other leaders in attendance in Buffalo (2002).

Photo Gallery

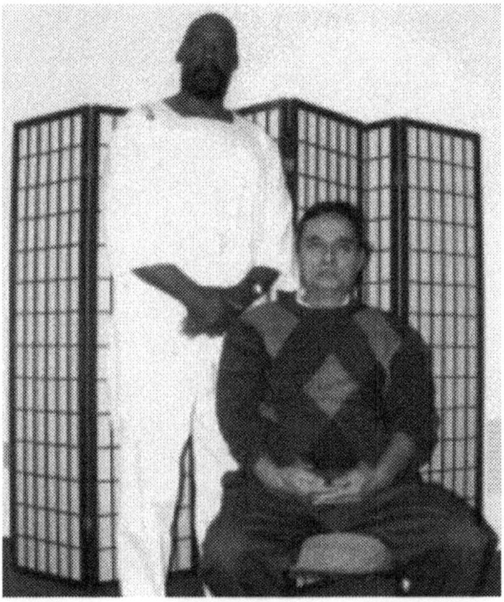

Dr. Mahn Saing is a trusted medical advisor an avid Tai Chi practitioner from Thailand from whom I have learned much about health and wellness. I am fortunate to have him as part of my team and class.

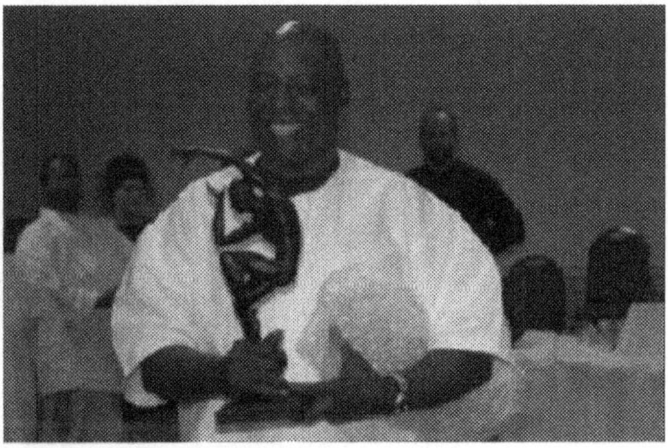

A surprise award given at the Black Family Conference in Louisville, Kentucky in March 2006
Photo courtesy of
RamImages.com

Photo Gallery

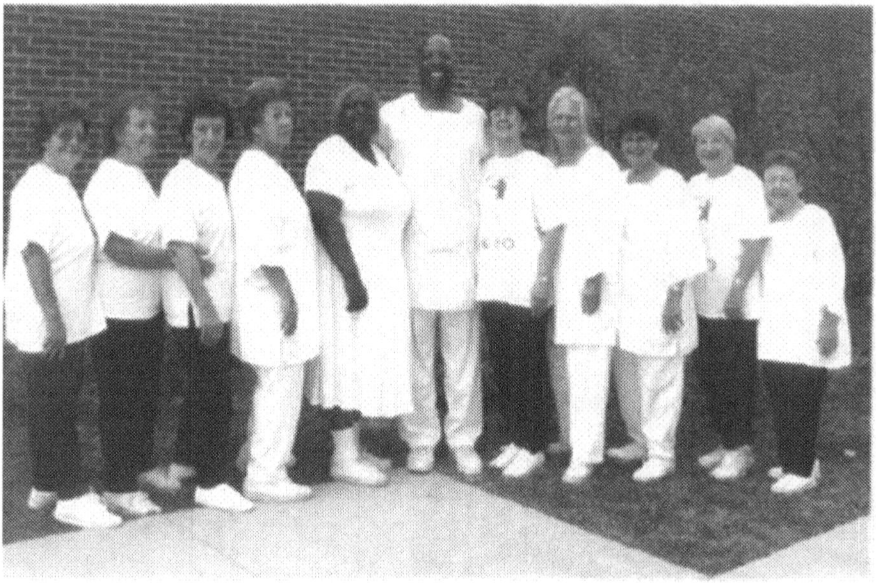

A pose with senior group after Tai Chi class

A memory lane shot preparing a student for a karate competition

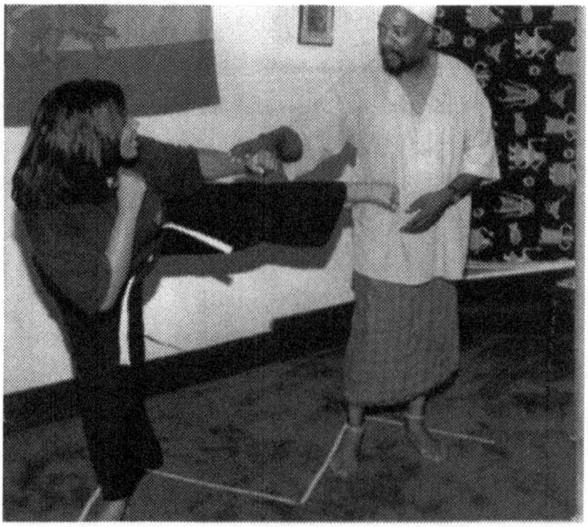

Photo Gallery

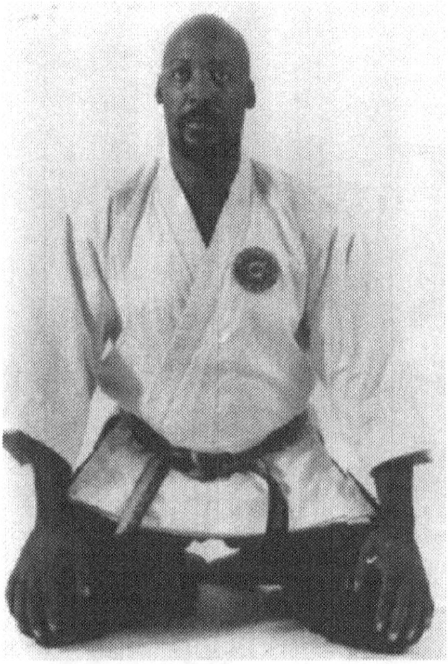

Karate served a very important purpose in my life

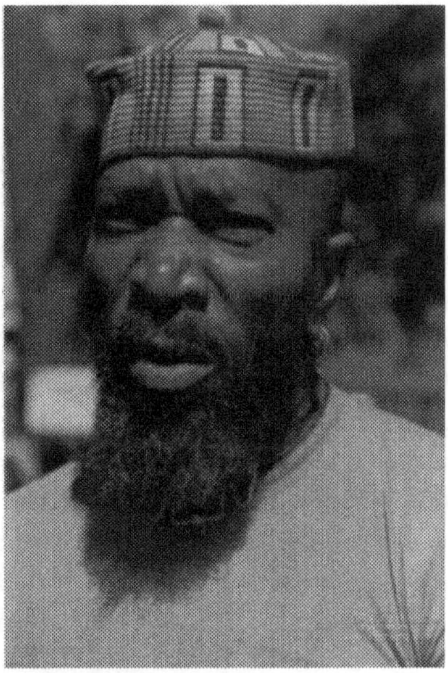

Brother Atu: a master drummer, woodcarver, storyteller, player of African musical instruments—you name it! He is also a master friend and encourager.

My mental, physical and spiritual health and well-being rest in ancient Afrikan principles that enhance and support the unity and growth of all people.

~Mfundishi Obuabasa Serikali

6

Tai Chi & Spirituality

"Open the doors and who'll come in? Who'll come in? Who'll come in?
Open the doors and who'll come in so early in the morning?…"

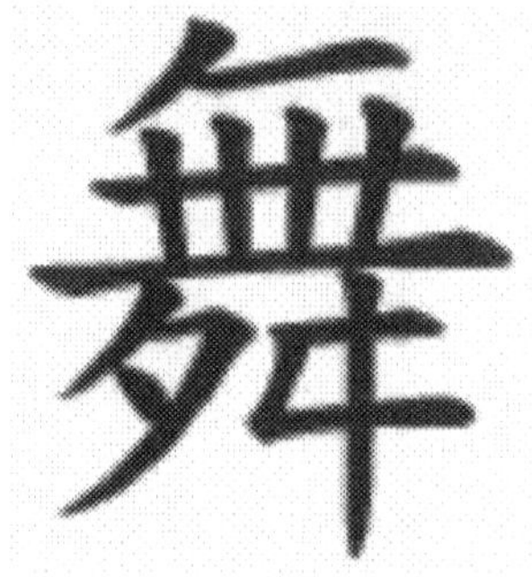

Wu (Dance)

Remember that little song from childhood? Actually, practicing Tai Chi is like opening a door to the self inside as I tap into my spirituality through focus and concentration. There is no attempt to coerce but rather to cooperate. I must emphatically state that Tai Chi is not a religion of any kind. Because the art is based on Taoist principles, some unfamiliar with the common threads of the different religions have tried to claim that practicing Tai Chi is anti-Christian. Because of the Eastern origins, those Christians may be concerned about an incompatible spirituality. This could not be further from the truth. A simple practice with profound results, Tai Chi focuses on the harmony among body, mind and spirit. Tai Chi is a way to feel good, re-energize the body and at the same time find inner calm and serenity—nothing more and nothing less. Tai Chi provides, not merely an experience, but the *significance* of that experience: not just a wild wind, but also a feeling for the *mystery* in the sound of that wind at night. As a tool to ideal living, Tai Chi cultivates spirituality in its higher levels beyond the concept of religion. An African-Asian proverb states, "There are many ways and by-ways that lead to one great highway." Indeed, the "quietness" of Tai Chi is ideal for spending time in the Presence of God. The following paragraph is an excerpt from *TAI CHI: Spiritual Martial Art* by William L. Pensky:

> The practice of Tai Chi has many purposes. For at least the last six hundred years, it has been a meditational form, a health practice, part of the Oriental system of martial arts, and an art the perfection of which—like any art—could be used to approach the Tao. In the final analysis, Tai Chi is a sacred dance. The movement, postures, and the connection between the two exist independently of the abilities of the performer, and call forth, when done correctly, a definite relationship between the performer and his understanding of the entirety of what he has learned and experienced. And as a sacred dance it is a prayer—a call for the evoking of the movement of the Tai Chi—the Grand Ultimate, the life force. A real prayer is not a petition for results but a position from which to see.

Pensky goes on to explain that this "quietness" or "watchfulness" is not violent but is serious because my real value to myself is at stake. I believe that the slow and steady movements of Tai Chi, often described as "stillness in motion", lift the happenings of everyday life out of the commonplace. The practitioner finds an exhilaration that comes from the complementary compatibility between breath and movement, inner and outer, *Yin* and *Yang*. More than any other of the martial arts, Tai Chi develops sensitivity to the power energy of the universe. It has been said that whatever is done each day is a prayer stemming from the spirituality inside. Indeed, the experiences we encounter in life, the people who come into our lives and those who leave our lives, the journeys taken, the passions explored, and the lessons learned all serve as tools that enable our spiritual nature to grow. I spend a great deal of time talking to my students about the need for spiritual enlightenment and how that basis produces the fertile ground for growth in the art of Tai Chi. When seeking balance, peace, harmony, cooperation and fewer stressful events in life, the real need is for spiritual growth. The Tai Chi instructor can assist the student by providing a different frame of reference that elevates the intensity of feeling to the spiritual process of awakening to soul realization. The student becomes more in tune with the natural flow all around as the instructor guides the student through the movements. The Tai Chi instructor helps to activate the *chi*, or vital energy, that lies deep within the student and with daily practice and development of proper breathing the student continues to build up the *chi* within.

Dr. Ronald L. Mann has explored this process of transference between the student and the instructor to some degree. In an article titled, *Activation: A Process of Spiritual Awakening*, he states that people experience spiritual awakening in a variety of ways. Furthermore, he continues, there is a psychological and spiritual occurrence between two people when spiritual consciousness is first ignited. He calls this process "activation" and notes that there are a variety of situations in which this spiritual dynamic can occur. We are accustomed to this phenomenon as it happens regularly in our various places of worship; however, this "activation" also occurs in Tai Chi. As the student begins to flow with the movements, the awareness of the higher self is brought from the subconscious to the conscious. However, a student can easily mistake the expanded, loving presence of the Tai Chi instructor as a personal expression of desire and connection. I believe that it is the responsibility of the Tai Chi instructor to keep the transference process healthy and balanced to effectuate maximum growth for the student. I do this by consistently imparting to my students the knowledge that the same energy found within and cultivated by daily practice is the same energy that connects to the "Ultimate Source" where there is love, peace, joy, bliss, light, and wisdom. In other words, it is not because of me but because of a much grander design. Remember that Tai Chi cultivates and fosters humility as we become aware. Tai Chi encourages the fulfillment of the individual person, yet also emphasizes that this goal should be achieved through moderate and natural ways of living.

Another virtue inherent in the practice of Tai Chi is patience. Too often we put the cart before the horse and try to force results as if the attainment was just another task to be accomplished. The desire to perfect the form very often drives the student to frustration. The one who does not develop spiritually will begin to feel that the instructor is not teaching the form fast enough or that the teacher no longer gives them the attention that they may have received when they first began. This is ego and I can't emphasize enough that a true practitioner of Tai Chi must "let go of ego." To no longer stroke the student's ego is all part of the training. I want the student to become rooted and to be able to withstand the chaos of the outer world because his/her inner world is in completeness or "bliss." Instead of accepting the *chi* and flowing with it, generally the student grows bored or disenchanted with learning Tai Chi. But, if the student does not work to deny the ego and focus on the lesson of the moment, the spiritual development of the student will be stifled and the student will not continue to mature in Tai Chi.

Mind. Body. Spirit. Can these entities be separated? No. Classic Martial Arts training teaches how to rise above the physical allowing the intellect to rule the body. Only when the physical nature has been placed under subjection to the mind will the mind be able to open up to spiritual realities. Practicing Tai Chi helps the student to maintain a perfect balance. Just as Tai Chi trains the enthusiast to move the physical body as one unit so, too, the practice of Tai Chi helps to maintain a perfect balance in this inseparable triune relationship. The physical activity is a way to achieve total oneness with ourselves and create harmony among body, mind and spirit. Strengthening the body, stimulating the mind, and freeing the soul of the yoke from years of repression are all nontransparent benefits of becoming a Tai Chi adept. The central concept of Tai Chi is that the mind, body, and spirit must work together to defeat an enemy-and enemies can be violent attackers, physical ailments, or mental illnesses. But what are some of the key element to being one in mind, body and spirit? There are three that I want my students to keep above all else: love, awareness and forgiveness/gratitude. This might very well be my take on faith, hope and charity but I want to stay true to the ancient ways of both the masters of Tai Chi and my ancestors. The old ways made it clear that to pass on knowledge is a privileged responsibility and it is up to the teacher to make sure that the student is able to receive it or else it must be withheld—even a bad disposition was, and still is, enough grounds to dismiss a potential student. Let me briefly discuss each of these three elements in turn.

In talking about love, it is always helpful to be reminded that there are three types as experienced in life: *agape, eros* and *phileo. Agape* love in its absolute form denotes the love of God—self-sacrificing and unconditional. In contrast there is self-centered *eros* love that wants something in return for what it gives. Also known as conditional love, erotic love easily exploits and takes the advantage for personal ends. Thirdly, there is *phileo* love shared between two people and commonly called "brotherly love." It is based on an inner communication and a mutual attraction between loving and being loved. Now, repeatedly practicing the movements of Tai Chi either heightens the process of loving self unconditionally or sets the student on this journey. The mind, body, and spirit have to become one in appreciating the true "self." There can be no fearful limits regarding what is achievable. Through the movements and continuous flow, Tai Chi takes the enthusiast to new heights of discovery. The practitioner becomes lost in the movements only to connect with self, the *Yin* and the *Yang*, and a renewed body. Obviously, only the unconditional, *agape* love begins to meet the requirements for love of self. And because we all understand the golden rule, only this kind of love fulfills the commission to love others. Discovering this unconditional love of the spirit brings spiritual balance and helps to improve the physical and mental well-being. Daily practice of Tai Chi from a center of unconditional love for self and others balances the spirit and helps to remove the layers of negative thinking and replace them with positive thoughts. Righteous loving promotes positive thinking; positive thinking promotes right feeling; right feeling promotes right action. Generally, relationships also improve as the practitioner begins to see others for who they are rather than for the person(s) they want them to be.

In the transformative process, we become the artists and the scientists of our lives. The transformed self has new tools, gifts, and sensibilities. Like the artist, the transformed self finds meaning and its own inescapable originality—"every life stands beneath its own star." Like the scientist, the transformed self experiments, speculates, invents and relishes the unexpected. Tai Chi enhances awareness and promotes in all of us the traits that abound in the creative person. That list would include, but is not limited to:

- whole-seeing
- freshness
- childlike perceptions
- playfulness
- a sense of flow
- risk-taking
- ability to focus attention in a relaxed manner
- ability to become lost in the object of contemplation
- ability to deal with many complex ideas at the same time
- willingness to diverge from the prevailing view
- access to preconscious material
- seeing what is there rather than what is expected

Here is the place where the eyes are opened and awareness bids the enthusiast to enter. When the student begins to awaken *chi* through the practice of Tai Chi, the paths for the natural flow must be clear and unblocked since any kind of tension will retard this natural flow. So, this transformative process depends on a level of awareness or consciousness that allows the true self to materialize. Since loving self includes not being afraid to be yourself, finding this level of consciousness becomes another part of the goal of transformation.

Although self-love sounds like a simple task there are many people, in fact, who are unhappy with themselves and find the task to be very difficult. For example, the pressure of looking thin outweighs the need to be healthy so self-love becomes conditional based on physical disciplines. If loving and accepting yourself is still a difficult task for you, then try the exercises included as Exhibit 5.1 at the end of this chapter. Love of self is the prerequisite to loving others and thereby achieving spiritual balance. Tai Chi can help to maintain spiritual balance and help to improve both physical and mental well-being. The rhythmic flowing movements of Tai Chi, which first appeal to enthusiasts of all ages, serve to build the inner self—the spiritual self. How is that spiritual self cultivated in Tai Chi? In the movements of Tai Chi one begins to love oneself unconditionally by placing no boundaries on the outer or inner self. Through the continuous flow of the movements, the practitioner is taken to new heights of discovery about the limitlessness of the flesh when motivated by spirit (intent). Daily practice of Tai Chi helps the practitioner to reach higher levels of consciousness and awareness.

The practice of Tai Chi can transport the practitioner to a level of awareness beyond the execution of the form. It is approaching the grand ultimate wherein becoming better at the art is eclipsed by becoming better as a person. The success of the external mastery of Tai Chi is only a reflection of the mastery of inner opponents. The exercise becomes the means to experiencing a personal potential greater than the physical achievement. This shift in awareness is a subtle benefit of practicing Tai Chi. Making a deep, soulful connection to life through the physical experience is a by-product of accepting the challenges within and being conscious of self as the opponent. The physical stimulation opens doors to the inner emotional concerns as well as the deep center of truth regarding life lessons about criticism, patience, crisis, loyalty, loss and many others. Indeed, only by conquering our self-imposed limitations can we move to higher levels of physical achievement. When the mind and body are in this open state, we are more receptive to personal growth and change without being defensive. As we move away from outer results, we begin to make discoveries about who we really are. There are many theories and schools of thought concerning the levels of consciousness. Author Ed Rabel states in this book, *Basic Spiritual Awareness*, that there are twelve levels. This thought is echoed by Paulson & Paulson in *Chakras, Auras and the New Spirituality*. There is not much written information pertaining to levels eight through twelve, but the first seven levels can be summarized as follows:

- Level 1: False Personality
- This is the lowest level of human existence
- Level 2: Man Asleep
- In this state one is walking with eyes open, yet still asleep or unaware of self and surroundings
- Level 3: Mechanical Existence

- Our creativity is not our own. We are fooled into thinking that our ideas are our own when, in fact, we have been programmed into how we should think, act and feel. We think we know ourselves, but we do not. Our thoughts linger on what others think of us or how others see us.
- Level 4: Man Remembering
- Something happens in our lives and we begin to remember by thinking for ourselves, defining ourselves and speaking for ourselves. This level can be likened to Simba's experience in the Disney movie, *The Lion King*. Rafiki, the monkey, continually hits Simba on the head to jar his memory! Later, the spirit of Simba's father tells him to remember who he is and reclaim his rightful place in the order of the universe. At this level we begin to realize that we are connected to a universal source. (To move from level 3 to level 4 we sometimes need a jolt on the head or something else to open our eyes and cause us to awaken.)
- Level 5: Man Awakening
- At this level we become more aware of our actions and the actions of others
- Level 6: Conscious Man
- Now our creativity and our energy is positive
- Level 7: Real Man
- Here we have reached conscious awareness of ourselves and our interactions with our surroundings

No matter what the religious experience, markers along the way that in some way correspond to these levels can roughly delineate a person's spiritual journey. Most people begin their journey floundering between Level 1 and Level 3. These levels comprise the negative attitudes, faults, and transgressions. At the awakening point leading to Level 4 one is said to be on the path or the way. Any time we become negative, continue to be negative, and are aware of being negative we fall back to the level of False Personality or Man Asleep or Mechanical Existence experiencing useless suffering along the way. Depression and feelings of hopelessness plague this relapse but we do not have to stay in this state. Tai Chi practice helps to keep the levels of consciousness open and pull us back up again. How? Remembering the basic principles of Tai Chi helps us to **physically** become still and find a quiet place free from noise and chaos. Then as we collect ourselves, we **mentally** turn within focusing on our center and concentrating on abdominal breathing. Finally, we **spiritually** gather our remembrance concerning who we are and whose we are as we connect with the Creator. Then we can move with the rhythm and the flow of life being consciously aware rather than metaphysically asleep.

All of the levels of awareness are within you, but your present level contains the greatest sense of "I AM" for you. Once you are aware of the power of consciousness, then it will be possible for you to shift your sense of "I AM" to a higher level. It is conceivable that parts of your sense of "I AM" are scattered across several levels and thus you may be confused and feel fragmented. But the act of centering yourself (through breathing and meditation) brings your sense of "I AM" into focus and allows you to choose to be aware on a higher level. If you are wise, you will set your center on a high level (above level three) but most people do not being comfortable at level one or two. In Tai Chi the aim is to wholly give the sense of "I AM" to the highest level of awareness possible.

I often tell my students that in practicing Tai Chi we are practicing in the spirit, not asleep, otherwise it would be mechanical. Tai Chi helps to center through breath and breathing. So when the knees begin to ache it is an awakening that we have neglected our bodies. Tai Chi is a call to get into the dynamic moment of life and turn off the mechanics. Move with the rhythm and flow. Discover which level of consciousness contains the greatest sense of "I AM" for you. You have the power to control your own sense of "I AM" for when you are awakened and aware of the power of consciousness then you can shift your sense of "I AM" from the lower to the higher levels. I urge students to set their center on a high level—above level three—because certain mental and emotional attitudes have the effect of draining a person's *chi*. One of these negative, draining attitudes that I often encounter is the attitude of being owed something: life owes better treatment; people owe more admiration; children owe more respect; parents owe larger allowances and more freedom; beloved partners owe more love; elderly parents are owed more visits; and the list goes on. Such beliefs act like poison to the soul and deplete vital energy at a rapid rate. If the mind harbors any thought of being wronged, it is impossible to let in the cleansing power of spirit and the richness of spiritual substance until the thought is cast out and forgiveness is in operation. As the slate is wiped clean of debts owed, the soul is cleansed and spiritual blockages are removed. Forgiveness creates new vital energy and greatly improves health allowing the *chi* to flow uninhibited. Gratitude takes us beyond our ego to the pathway that does not squander and waste our vital, health-improving energy. Holding on to these negative feelings may lead to illness, disease and even death because the flow of the vital energy has been blocked from bringing health and peace of mind. In the book *Heal Your Body: The Mental Causes for Physical Illness and The Metaphysical Ways to Overcome Them* author Louise L. Hay covers the many blockages we may encounter along with the powerful, yet simple, ways to regain our physical and spiritual ground. I often teach a simpler tactic: consider what you owe to others. Considering what we ought to be doing for others and what we owe to our Creator further enlarges the attitude of gratitude. I believe that each of us owes a cosmic debt of love and gratitude. By assuming such a debt we place ourselves in the healthiest of all positions possible for a human being because it places us right in the heart of the infinite *agape* consciousness.

Continual practice of Tai Chi will bring forth whatever is the dominant energy—positive or negative. That is why any negativity must go. Loving self and acceptance of self are of utmost importance as Tai Chi helps to tune in to the inner dialog and practices focusing on the inner awareness. It is a way to the greater awakening of the true self and the achievement of enlightenment. What is enlightenment? It is the freedom of choice at 360 degrees achieved by daily tuning in to our inner text and posing the right questions: "What do I want now?" "What decisions am I making now?" "What am I doing now?" The amount of time it takes to become enlightened depends on the individual. Each journey is different and each person must go at a pace appropriate for him/her. The timing must be right, so follow your own heart and intuitive sense. Consider the following story shared with me by my teacher:

> ***There was once a rich king who had four wives. He loved the fourth wife the most and adorned her with rich robes and treated her to the finest delicacies. He gave her nothing but the best. He also loved the third wife very much and showed her off to neighboring kingdoms. However, he feared that one day she would leave him for another. He also loved the second wife. She was his confidante and was always kinds, considerate and patient with him. Whenever the King faced a problem he would confide in her to help him get through the difficult times. The King's first wife was a very loyal partner and had made great contributions in maintaining his wealth and kingdom. However, he did not love the first wife and although she loved him deeply, he hardly took notice of her.***
>
> ***One day, the King fell ill and he knew that his time was short. Thus he asked the fourth wife, "Since I have loved you the most, endowed you with the finest clothing and showered great care over you, now that I am dying, will you follow me and keep me company?"***
> ***"No way!" replied the 4th wife and she walked away without another word.***

The sad King asked the 3rd wife, "Since I have loved you all my life, now that I am dying will you follow me and keep me company?"
"No!" replied the 3rd wife. "Life is too good! When you die I am going to remarry!" His heart sank and turned cold.
He then asked the second wife, "Since I have always turned to you for help and you've always been there for me, when I die will you follow me and keep me company?"
"I'm sorry; I can't help you out this time!" replied the 2nd wife. "At the very most, I can only send you to your grave." Her answer came like a bolt of thunder and the King was devastated.
Then a voice called out: "I'll leave with you and follow you no matter where you go."
The King looked up and there was his first wife. She was so skinny because she suffered from malnutrition. Greatly grieved, the King said, "I should have taken better care of you when I had the chance!"

* * *

In truth, we all have four wives in our lives:

- *Our fourth wife is our body. Not matter how much time and effort we lavish in making it look great, it will leave us when we die.*
- *Our third wife is our possessions, status, and wealth. When we die, it will all go to others.*
- *Our second wife is our family and friends. No matter how much they have been there for us, the furthest they can stay by us is up to the grave.*
- *Our first wife is our soul, often neglected in pursuit of wealth, power and pleasures of the ego. However, our soul is the only thing that will follow us wherever we go.*

Practicing Tai Chi is a way to the greater awakening of the Self. It is a path to authentic living where our inner world is truthfully reflected in our outer expression. For many, Tai Chi is incorporated into their daily lives as a means for the *chi* to heal the mind, body and spirit. A great amount of time is spent to keep the body in shape and to sustain mental capacity, but the soul—the essence, the spirit—is very often neglected. So, cultivate, strengthen and cherish it now! It is your greatest gift to offer the world…keeping connected with your soul is called ***harmony***. Daily affirm that you are a whole, complete being at one with God and having access to God's Divine ideas at all times. In so doing you will become fit both externally and internally. Consider the exercises and activities on the following pages to help start you on your way.

Exercises for Practicing Self-Acceptance

1. Mirror Self Analysis

   Stand before a mirror, alone, paper and pencil at hand. Draw a line down the center of the page. On the left hand side of the page write, "This is what I accept about myself." (I did not use the word 'love' here.) On the other side write, "This is what I do not accept about myself." Then hold an honest and open discourse with that image in the mirror.

   See yourself on many different levels of reality, from the highest to the lowest, from the most mature to the most immature, from the sweetest to the harshest, from the most loving to the angriest you have ever been. Allow yourself to experience the love, the compassion, the hate, the rage, the jealously and the sacrifice. Begin to take note of how you judge yourself, how you disbelieve your lovingness, how you take pride in your self-censuring.

   None of this is to be done harshly because there has been enough of that. But do it with an eye to truth. Notice how the shame you feel when you truly love yourself is heartbreaking. Decide that you have come to learn love because you cannot love another more than you love yourself and you cannot love God more than you love another. Hold this dialogue with yourself in the mirror for at least ten minutes, more if you like, but at least ten minutes. Then close your eyes and see yourself bathed in the radiant light of love. Accept it. Let it come through your pores. See yourself bathed in love every minute of every day for you are love.

2. "Hello me, this is Me."

   Reacquaint your lower self with your Higher Self. Go within into your silence. Envision yourself entering a room. No one is there with you. Suddenly, across the room, you perceive yourself as you really are, in your inner beauty. Allow yourself to make your acquaintance, tenderly lovingly. Now take you Self by the hand. Bring your Self back with you. Keep your Self close to you for the rest of your life. The Self you have just met has been waiting to be noticed throughout your life. Once you have learned who you are, you will begin to realize that it matters very little what anyone else things. As you emerge from behind the mask of your personality, see yourself as unabashedly giving love and delight, smiling all the time. See yourself with the divine task of spreading light and love wherever you are…let it be contagious.

3. Erasing Your Physical Boundaries

   Close your eyes and envision the outline of your physical body as though it were drawn with a very dark pencil. (Be faithful to the shape of your body.) This outline identifies your personality-ego structure.

   Now envision a large erase and allow it to begin to erase the lines of the physical body. (Note the portions that prove move stubborn than others to erase. This information is useful for later self-inquiry.) When you reach the top of your head, do an exceptionally good job of erasing that area. Do not resist and accept whatever happens. This will take some time. Allow the consciousness of Self to expand. You have now challenged the illusion of human physical experience. Depending on how courageous you have been in erasing, you have permitted yourself to expand far beyond that line of physical identity. Now you can embrace your whole Self. Live in the Eternal Now.

Activities for Creating "Smiling Energy"

1. Activities for expectancy, hope and self-affirmation
   a. Read a book
   b. Write a book
   c. Begin a research project
   d. Adopt a pet, friend, or family
   e. Do needlepoint or another craft
   f. Begin gardening
   g. Begin Tai Chi
2. Activities for laughter, letting go, going beyond yourself
   a. Share a joke or ridiculous thought
   b. Make funny faces or weird noises
   c. Play games
   d. Play with a child
   e. Go to the amusement park and ride the roller coasters
   f. Learn to be a clown
   g. Practice Tai Chi

3. Activities for reflection, growth, expanding your universe
    a. Dream
    b. Think
    c. Take a trip inside
    d. Take a trip outside
    e. Keep a journal
    f. Do nothing
    g. Breathe
    h. Feel your feelings
    i. Move or dance
    j. Watch stones grow
    k. Watch and listen to the trees
    l. Walk a labyrinth
    m. Continue Practicing Tai Chi
4. Activities for your body, strength, vitality
    a. Observe it
    b. Get in the water
    c. Practice good nutrition
    d. Get enough sleep
    e. Dress up
    f. Exercise
    g. Get exposed to good sounds and smells
    h. Pamper it
    i. Practice Tai Chi more

Keep your thoughts positive because your thoughts become your words.
Keep your words positive because your words become your behaviors.
Keep your behaviors positive because your behaviors become your habits.
Keep your habits positive because your habits become your values.
Keep your values positive because your values become your destiny.

~Chinese proverb

Soft and weak overcome hard and strong.
...And
He who stands of tiptoe is not steady.
He who strides cannot maintain the pace.

-Lao Tzu (Tao Te Ching)

7

Tai Chi Technique

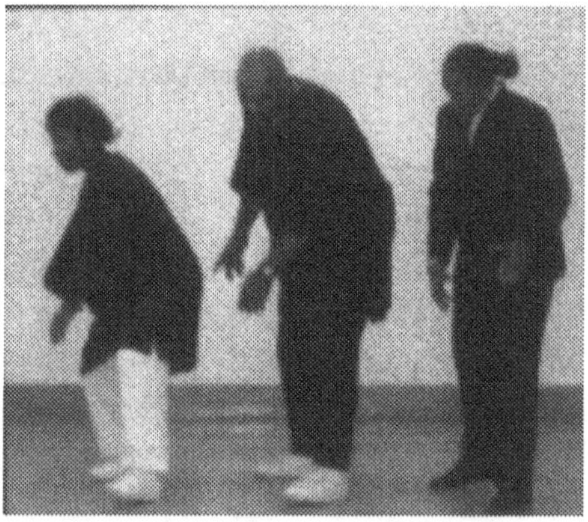

More students receive instruction

Most of the styles of Tai Chi have created an abbreviated form, between twenty and forty movements, that allows for quicker learning and shortened practice time. Although greater emphasis is placed on the Tai Chi form, or set of movements, as related to maintaining good health, I agree with those who point out that learning the form without any understanding of the meaning of the movements serves to create an empty, tactically incorrect form. By this I mean that the martial aspect of Tai Chi is at the core of every movement. As Pensky states, "Like so many other oriental arts, it has become enormously popular in this country, primarily as a physical exercise. But this is certainly not its deepest meaning, and I believe that when we concern ourselves with the practices of other cultures, it behooves us to use care and respect." Tai Chi consists of separate strong and powerful movements that are connected together into a specific order.

While the solo form may appear to be separate from any martial application, it is the foundation for further study of the combat aspects of Tai Chi. There are, however, no belts or degrees in Tai Chi. Weapons and partner practice complete it as a competition sport and system of self-defense. Foremost to remember is that Tai Chi is a tool designed to generate *chi* and to actualize, mobilize and motivate the movement of this *chi* in its course around the body throughout the meridians through which it flows. Doing this brings about harmony and balance and empowerment to fight. Generally speaking, the average Tai Chi student today is not interested in learning a fighting technique. So, although every posture that is learned by the student does have a martial application, the mastery of the understanding of that martial application is of secondary importance. I believe that Grandmaster Cheng Man-Ching and those before him would readily adapt their teaching to focus on health for the greater advancement of the art. Therefore, I can not agree with those who believe that focusing on the health aspect in any way creates a weak substitute. In the history of martial arts, there have been those who thought that the internal arts would die because they did not look strong and sometimes external techniques were added to make them appear more credible. Fortunately, Tai Chi has had great masters to show that it is credible both as a martial art and as an aid to good health.

The training of combat skills in Tai Chi is in no way separate from the training for health and relaxation: slowly and without over exertion. Those students who do wish to learn the self defense aspect of the art will learn how to apply the principles of the art in order to divert an aggressor's attack and launch a counter attack. Students will train with partners to learn how to sense the direction of an attack and, to quote the classic teaching of the art, to "use one ounce to deflect a thousand pounds." In self-defense, Tai Chi movements should be natural and relaxed. The training allows power to be harnessed and issued from any position, giving way to attack and counterattacking with great efficiency and power. This harnessing of *chi* allows a tremendous amount of power to be generated with no windup or display of focus. Combined with heightened sensitivity gained from pushing hands, this gives the Tai Chi adept what is needed to control the situation. Generally speaking, one has to be truly expert to use most forms of Tai Chi effectively in self-defense, but it is a level of achievement that is not totally out of reach for the dedicated and conscientious student. However, to reach a good standard of martial skill will take a dedication to solo practice and physically demanding training. While it may take the average person many years of practice and study to utilize Tai Chi as a fighting art, the health benefits for the body of doing Tai Chi on a regular basis happen much quicker. The most important approach to the art, whether you simply wish to improve your health or become a martial artist, is patience. My focus in this chapter will be on general Tai Chi technique; I will leave the more detailed martial instruction for individual teachers to cover.

Now in China and worldwide, literally millions of citizens practice Tai Chi every day; some singularly, some in groups numbering into the hundreds, some with swords, some with large red fans. Tai Chi as part of a health regimen is practiced daily by millions because it requires no special equipment. The Yang long form consists of one hundred eight postures, many of which are repetitions of thirty-seven basic movement patterns. It can be practiced in a relatively small area either indoors or outdoors. The graceful form has a slow-motion, dance-like quality that gradually builds *chi*. It is the emphasis on soft overcoming hard and internal *chi* power overpowering external physical power that justifies Tai Chi as being the "grand ultimate" form suitable for healthy exercise. What are the most important points for progressing in Tai Chi? I would say they are: proper instruction, perseverance, and quality, not quantity, of movement. The goal of the exercise is to arrive at a balancing of the movement with no excess muscular activity or tension, keeping the body balanced on the spine, the spinal column pivoted at a point in its center of gravity so that at any given moment all the parts of the body are properly balanced. Tai Chi can be properly learned only by paying attention to the control of each muscle group to rid the body of stiffness and rigidity and achieve proper balance. The muscles should never be tensed to create force and power because force and power must be internally restrained and never be externally revealed.

As we practice it today, Tai Chi is often described as a moving form of yoga and meditation combined. What does Tai Chi have to offer that yoga does not? Perhaps it is as the saying goes, "Not the lotus, but the essence of the lotus." There are a number of forms (sometimes called "sets") that consist of movements. Many may have originally derived from the martial arts and the movements of animals; however, in Tai Chi they are performed slowly, softly and gracefully with smooth and even transitions between them. The movements are performed in this manner to generate and circulate the vital energy—*chi*—within the body thereby enhancing the health and vitality of the practitioner. This is achieved because the movements alternate in a definite and steady rhythm between yielding receptivity (*Yin*) and forceful creation (*Yang*). According to Traditional Chinese Medicine (TCM), *chi* circulates in patterns that are closely related to the nervous and vascular systems and behaves in accordance with those ideas connected with the practices of acupuncture and other oriental healing arts. At the end of the Tai Chi practice, the *chi* has made one complete revolution throughout the body's meridian system. One complete performance of the Tai Chi form, if done correctly, generates the flow of the *chi* throughout the body in its revitalizing capacity as it would move in one full twenty-four-hour period. Another aim of Tai Chi is to foster a calm and tranquil mind, focused on the precise execution of the movements. It is not an exercise of will and determination, but an exercise of attention and observation. The goal is to integrate physical form with concentration meaning that the aim is to guide and control the movements of the body through the thoughts. Using visualization is an indispensable aid in achieving agreement between what the mind is thinking and what the body is doing. While doing Tai Chi, the mind must be quiet ad peaceful in order to fully concentrate on the movements and avoid distractions. In addition, Tai Chi helps to increase body awareness. The graceful movements gently increase the body's range of motion while exercising the internal organs. In learning the postures and connecting each posture in a specific manner, the practitioner learns how to control the body and mind in harmony. Having learned all of the postures, the Tai Chi form is then refined through meditative practice. As relaxation and alignment improve, the practitioner returns repeatedly to the beginning to reach a higher level. In this manner, the form develops into a natural state for the practitioner that merely copying a teacher's form cannot produce. After being able to sense the flow of *chi* in the body, the mind can begin to guide the *chi* while directing the body and its movements at will. In this way, the mind and body will reach harmony.

What is the position of the body during Tai Chi practice? First, practice time is where the slowness of Tai Chi is indispensable and cannot be underestimated! Learning to control muscles is the difficulty in the beginning but necessary to adequately learn all the nuances of each movement. Therefore, the beginner **must** take deliberate care to execute each movement as slowly as possible. Students should learn one movement at a time, systematically. The most important concept for both students and instructors to remember is not to rush through training but to be thorough. Those who try to learn too much too fast do not assimilate well and have a poor foundation for future learning. Without the confidence fostered by that solid foundation, they are apt to get sloppy and become confused as to techniques and application. When this happens, it is very difficult to attain the proper clarity of mind. Therefore, the structure of the training should be gradual and thorough, for after learning one step well the student progresses naturally to the next. Next, the student must learn to flow—attain continuity of movement with a constant rate. Ideally, the moves will flow continuously and without pause, from one to another, in an even exchange of postures. Pausing to adjust the feet or body position during the form is unacceptable although necessary in the beginning phase. To achieve the desired smooth pace the practitioner must also develop the discipline of total consciousness while doing the movements. My teacher suggested imagining the movements as they would appear under a strobe light. By visualizing a series of stills within each movement, the form becomes internalized and semi-automatic removing conscious effort from the routine.

In Tai Chi there should be an overall impression of relaxed yet alert energy that surrounds and moves swiftly through the body. "Relaxed yet alert" may seem contradictory, but think for a moment about standing in a swimming pool with the water level approximately neck-high. As a matter of fact, the body should appear to move as though moving through water rather than flesh and bone moving through weightless air. Imagine that the air actually takes on the quality of water and the body is aware of the resistance of the air around it. The body itself feels light but more importantly mental lightness (intent) is used to control the lightness of the movements. Here the student has arrived at the second stage of the development of relaxation where the training of the thoughts and the mind are concerned with the execution of the form as it has been learned. While performing the movements, the mind keeps alive the questions within: "Am I relaxed?" Am I moving from my center of gravity?" In other words, during the first stage of development the thought is the leader, learning the sequence of the movements. In the second stage, the body has learned the sequence and now the mind must be attentive, follow and question its relationship to the body to achieve balanced movements. Finally, during the third stage the concentration of the mind is upon the application and the understanding of the presence of the opponent in the practice of the form. Understanding the function of each movement aids the learning process. Too many students learn abstract ballet like movements that have no real meaning to them, causing confusion and lack of precision. But by understanding the applications it is easier to remember the correct performance of each technique. I find it helpful to demonstrate the defensive and offensive applications of the form movements as the student learns each. When the students know the meaning of the movements, I can see correct performance become more internalized through diligent practice.

Not until the student reaches this third stage where there is no thought but the movement will *chi* be generated. This develops from the stillness fostered by practice and by not letting too much energy escape through shifting eyes or an open mouth. Remember that Tai Chi brings together the spirit, intent, internal energy and the body to form a superior skill. Over time the student should strive to harmonize the spirit with the intent, the intent with the internal energy, and the internal energy with physical strength. According to *The Essence of Tai Chi*, the internal energy must be expended and vibrated like the beat of a drum while the spirit is condensed in toward the center of the body.

Movement in Tai Chi is non-linear or circular as created by Chang San-feng so many years ago. All movements, no matter how small, must be controlled by the intent. Physiologically, movement comes from the joints that connect the bones and the surrounding muscle groups. The use of circular movements intrinsically generates more force than linear motion but practice is necessary to develop natural movements without tension. The range of motion of the joints is increased as they become more agile and flexible utilizing these circular motions.

Although in the initial stages the arms and hands appear to lead the body, ultimately the circular movements of the arms and hands follow the body powered from the waist. The waist is the power source and all movements will appear to be emanating from the waist and flow outward to the fingers in a smooth, uninterrupted flow. In good Tai Chi, if you carefully watch the shoulders and arms, you will see that only one joint moves at a time. This movement will be performed so smoothly that it appears to be a continuous flow. There are no exotic hand and finger formations in Tai Chi and movements should not look sleepy, limp, and listless.

With the exception of the beginning of the form, the body weight will never be equally distributed on both legs for any length of time. This is sometimes referred to as being double-weighted and is definitely prohibited in Tai Chi. (This does not apply when performing breathing or flexibility exercises based on some of the Tai Chi movements.) Most often, however, the terms 'emptiness' or 'fullness' are used to describe this principle in motion (also called being single-weighted). The feet are placed firmly in contact with the earth before weight is shifted to the front or back, and the knees never extend beyond the toes during a lunge. The *chi* energy is generated in the feet, issued through the legs, controlled in the waist, and driven out through the hands and fingers. The upper body, moving as one unit controlled by the waist, is carried seemingly riding above the hips. Weight is carried so that it presses directly into the earth through one foot at all times. The planting of the feet allows the body to be stable and rooted and for the upper and lower parts of the body to be mutually coordinated. Allowing the major joints to be relaxed, loosened, and exercised also helps to coordinate the upper and lower body.

Proper body alignment is a significant aspect of learning Tai Chi. Practicing poor body mechanics will stress the joints and cause chronic joint problems, especially in the knees. Unlike learning from a book or video, an instructor will repeatedly correct students with improper knee and back alignment. Why is it so important to have proper alignment in practicing good Tai Chi? The knee is a hinge joint, which moves well in only one plane of motion—front to back. The knees should never be twisted as such movement only leads to both short-term and long-term problems. Also, they should be in natural alignment with the toes, never going beyond the toes. Likewise, the back should be straight and never bent in order to avoid later back problems and to attain good balance with the head held high with a feeling of energy suspending it from above. The body should be light and relaxed, but not dead or limp—that is not what is meant here by relaxation. All stiffness and strength must be emptied from the upper torso and should sink to the soles of the feet, yet the body should feel alive and full of vigor. Overall, there should be a great impression of being well centered. Each movement should appear to give off waves of deep, quiet strength without any feeling of restrained tension, although the body will still be erect, yet relaxed, light and agile while appearing to almost float. At the same time, the body, steps, hands, and eyes must move in one complete direction through focus and intent.

Try to visualize the various parts of the body as follows:

- Head—kept vertical creating an upward suspension as if a plumb line dropped from the heavens through the crown point
- Face—looking calm and serene (no grimacing, teeth-gritting, etc.)
- Eyes—focused forward looking to infinity just over the forward hand, but not glaring
- Teeth/Lips—closed with the tongue rolled upward toward the back of mouth to keep the mouth moist
- Chin—slightly tucked
- Neck—relaxed
- Shoulders/Arms—rounded, loosened, never tensed
- Elbows—down
- Palms—when kept open, fingers slightly spread and extended
- Fist—in punching, the closed fist is kept perpendicular and not parallel to the ground
- Chest—hollow, slightly concave, relaxed and not expanded
- Back—rounded

- Waist—relaxed, sunk down, flexible
- Spine—straight with slight curve forward
- Coccyx—slightly tucked
- Hips—relaxed to support all turns with groin open and round
- Knees—bent, aligned with toes but never extending beyond toes during a stance; never twisted in or out over the instep or outside edge of the feet
- Legs—strong support for knees
- Feet—firmly in contact with the earth before weight is shifted to front or back; the front foot will point in the direction faced at the completion of each move; toes relaxed

Coordinated with all of the movements of the body is proper breathing. Explosive exhalations or exotic breathing methods are not a part of Tai Chi. Although it may be regulated, breathing should be natural—in through the nose, down to the lower abdomen, and out through the mouth. The breath should not be labored or held during the execution of any part of the form. It is very important to teach proper breathing as well as mental imagery in coordination with the movements from the very beginning. I find that students who are proficient with breathing techniques progress quicker and possess greater fluidity of movement than those who are not. If a practitioner is winded after finishing the form, something is wrong.

In the practice of Tai Chi self-discipline and structure are key ingredients. Remember that 'a journey of a thousand miles begins with one step' is an adage worth considering.

Nothing happens until something moves.

-Albert Einstein

8

Tai Chi and the Seven Golden Movements

Those who have not yet learned the whole Tai Chi form may practice movement exercises instead. In essence, these exercises are based loosely on the grace, fluidity, slowness and softness of Tai Chi. You will recall from our earlier discussions that every family of Tai Chi has closely guarded secrets that have been traditionally held within the families. Years ago my great brother and friend, Nganga Mfundishi Tolo-Naa, showed me the seldom seen *Secret Family Style* of the Yang Family Tai Chi as it was taught to him. It is still the most valued possession of the Yang family itself, and to this day it has never been committed to public print or record of any kind. So powerful and energizing is this style, that prior to its being performed, it requires a series of warm-up exercises that constitute, if practiced faithfully, a complete exercise system for health and longevity. As necessary as the ballet bar is to classical ballet—as necessary as the piano scales to a concert virtuoso—so, too, are the basic warm-ups to the *Secret Family Style*, the foundation for what is to follow. This series of exercises has been named ***The Seven Golden Movements.*** There are enough instructional videos and chapters in various books describing the movements of the various forms. Because these exercises can complement any style or stand on their own, I have chosen to use them as the basis for this chapter. Like Hua Tuo so many years ago and Einstein in more recent history, I believe in the intrinsic value of movement—specifically as it relates to health. If you never desire to master any of the Tai Chi forms, I believe that this basic series of exercises will provide you a way with which to live your life to the fullest, traveling your own path, enjoying good health, and serenity far into your golden years. If you are unfamiliar with Tai Chi, you would benefit from learning a basic form before attempting to follow the movements described in this section. It is best to know and adhere to the ten principles described below before adopting any movements for your health regimen.

Before we discuss the movements, I want to restate the fact that the body center (or *dan tian*) is the power point in the body for all movement. Finding this center, in your body and your mind, is of major importance. Throughout the history of Tai Chi and irrespective of the form or series of exercises practiced, there has always been one common denominator. It is called principle. Without the strict adherence to principle, Tai Chi would simply be empty form. The characteristics of good Tai Chi can be summarized by the following ten essential principles. Observing these essentials will keep the Tai Chi practitioner well within the framework of good Tai Chi. With consistent practice, your center will become very familiar to you. These Ten Principles of Tai Chi can be summarized as follows:

First principle—Hang the head
Hang the head from the crown as if suspended from a string above. The neck should be straight but not stiff so as to facilitate the flow of both breath and blood. The tongue should be touching the palate and breathing through the nose should be deep and natural. The energy at the top of the head should be light and sensitive.

Second principle—Sink the chest
Sink or hollow the chest allowing it to be naturally concave. Also raise the back and tuck the pelvis. This will allow the breath, the *chi*, to sink to the diaphragm or *dan tian*. Never breathe from the chest alone.

Third principle—Use the mind not force
Use intent not strength as the mind directs movement. You must practice using the mind to move the body instead of mundane strength. The mind must guide the movements of the body allowing yourself to relax completely so as not to impede the free flow of blood and breath between the sinew and bone.

Fourth principle—Sink shoulders and elbows
Let the shoulders sink and elbows drop downwards as if they are very heavy. If they are raised, they create tension in the body.

Fifth principle—Unity in the internal and external

Tai Chi also trains the body's spirit. Some say it is the essence of the art. The mind must move the spirit. Combine the internal and external as the spirit directs the physical. When the mind is able to raise the body's spirit, then the movements become light and nimble instead of heavy and clunky.

Sixth principle—Empty and full or *Yin* and *Yang*

This is basic to all Tai Chi. When the weight of the entire body is resting on the right leg, then the right leg is said to be full and the left leg empty and vice versa. So, differentiate full and empty so as not to be double weighted. When you can separate full and empty, you will be able to turn lightly and quickly. Without this principle, your steps will be heavy and slow and you will be off-balance.

Seventh principle—Unity between upper and lower body

Combine the upper and lower body and move as one unit. All motion should be rooted in the feet, released through the legs, controlled by the waist and pressed through the hand in one continuous flow.

Eighth principle—Seek slowness in movement

Unlike normal exercise where at the conclusion a person's energy is spent and they are out of breath, Tai Chi uses stillness to control movement; therefore the slower you move the better and stronger you perform. Understanding this principle will give you the real meaning of the art. Seek stillness in motion resulting in calm mind.

Ninth principle—Relax the waist

The waist is the axis of the entire body. The ability to changes between full and empty comes from a loose waist. If the waist is relaxed, the power is allowed to sink to the feet affording stability in movement.

Tenth principle—Continuity without interruption

Tai Chi should appear as a ballet throughout the entire form. Each move is completed without interruption and when one move ends another begins in continuous flowing strength. There is no vulnerability in good Tai Chi form—no break in the action. When there is a break in the body, there is a break in the mind. At that point, there is weakness. Tai Chi Chuan is like a great river in its continuous flow. Movements must be continuous like 'reeling silk'.

As you are probably deeply committed to raising families and achieving career goals, you face various day-to-day challenges and seek to find ways of dealing with them, both internally and externally. I mentioned earlier that the healing movement of *chi* starts first at the base and continues to move upward and outward making a complete circuit of the body. Indeed, every movement of the Tai Chi form takes *chi* to some part of the body. This particular moving meditation of Tai Chi's *Seven Golden Movements* provides specific coping mechanisms with which to deal with life in the modern world. I present it here as taught to me by my brother, Nganga Mfundishi Tolo-Naa, as his teacher, Professor Huo Chi-Kwang, taught it to him.

Preparation:

1. Stand with your feet together and knees slightly bent.

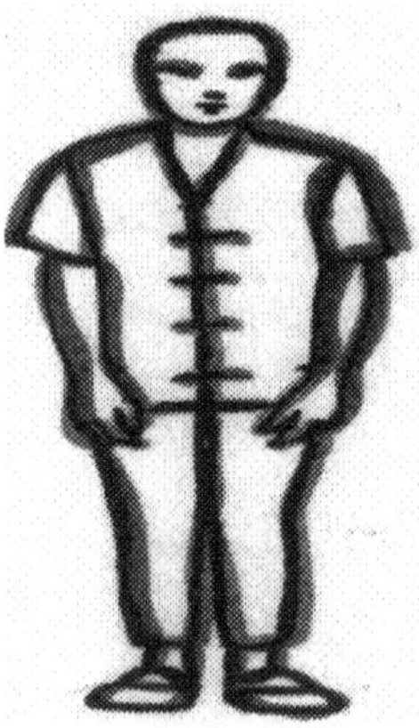

2. Place your hands at your sides.
3. Hang your head lightly as if from a string through the crown from above.
4. Place the tip of your tongue at the top of your palate behind your teeth.
5. Keep your mouth closed.
6. Relax and focus, breathing deeply.

Benefit:

This initial stance common to all Tai Chi forms gently gathers the energy to the *dan tian*, or body center, properly aligns the posture and calms the mind for the commencement of the exercise. It is here that mind, body and spirit are invoked as one to perform the movements.

Movement 1: Hold the Ball

1. Bend both knees.
2. Transfer all of your weight to the left leg.
3. Pick up your right heel.
4. Scribe a line shoulder width to the right.
5. Place your right foot down toe first.
6. Transfer your weight onto both legs evenly.

7. Place your hands in front of your thighs.
8. Slowly raise your arms to shoulder height and shoulder width.
9. Shift weight back and turn fingers to meet without touching.
10. Sit and hold the ball.

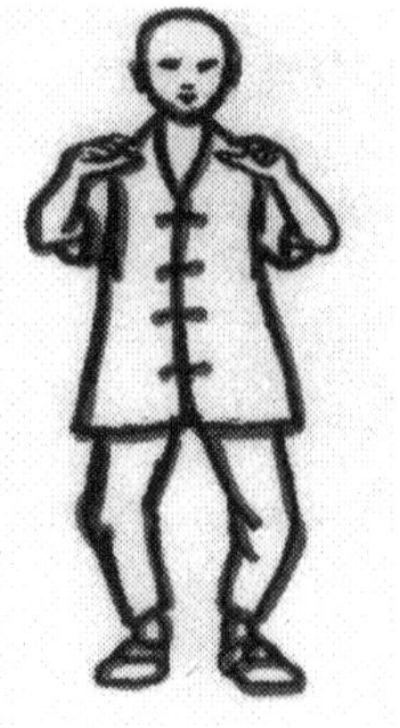

Benefit:

Holding the Ball is called 'the posture of love' and is most beneficial in strengthening the heart muscle. Although heart disease is the number one killer in the west, it is almost non-existent in China and this meditative posture is included in almost all of the various Tai Chi exercise regimens. In addition, this posture opens the rib cage to increase lung capacity and add incredible strength to the leg and thigh muscles, all of which supports the internal organs.

Movement 2: Bending Forward

1. From the end of **Hold the Ball**, straighten the arms and fingers.
2. Stand up and as your body comes up, let your arms go down in front of your body.
3. Shift your weight forward.
4. From here, look down and go down slowly and completely relaxed without forcing a stretch.
5. Let your body go down until it stops itself.
6. When your body stops, look backward with your head between your legs.
7. Reverse the arc by bringing your head back.
8. Slowly raise your body from the lower back using the same speed coming up as you did going down.
9. When your body straightens itself, transfer your weight back to your heel.
10. Tuck your pelvis and sit with hands in front of thighs.

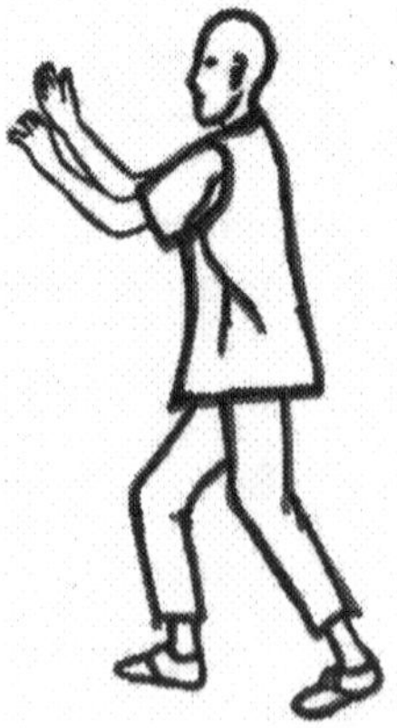

Repeat the entire sequence a second time:

1. Stand up.
2. Shift the weight forward.
3. Again, look down and go down completely relaxed (do not force a stretch).
4. Let the body go down until it stops itself.
5. When the body stops by itself, again look backwards between legs with your head.
6. Reverse the arc when it is complete.
7. Slowly raise the body up: same speed going down, same speed coming up.
8. As your body straightens out, again, shift weight back onto the heel.
9. Tuck your pelvis and sit.

Now repeat the entire sequence a third and final time:

1. Stand up.
2. Shift the weight forward.
3. Look down and go down without forcing the stretch.
4. Go down until your body stops itself.
5. Look back between your legs.
6. Reverse the arc of your head.
7. Come back up slowly—like drawing silk.
8. When your body straightens itself, shift your weight back onto your heels.
9. At the same time, raise both of your arms to shoulder width and shoulder height.
10. Sit and hold the ball.

Benefit:

This movement promotes a healthy, flexible spine. Think what it could mean to a person who spends dozens of stressful hours and weeks sitting at a computer terminal. Money spent on medication for lower back pain could float the national debt and think of what those pain killers are doing to our liver and pancreas. Don't pop pills is the key.

Movement 3: Golden Phoenix Rising

1. Straighten the arms and fingers.
2. From here, shift your weight to the left.
3. Bring your right toe in halfway.
4. Turn your waist slightly to the right, sit back on your left leg and bring your arms down

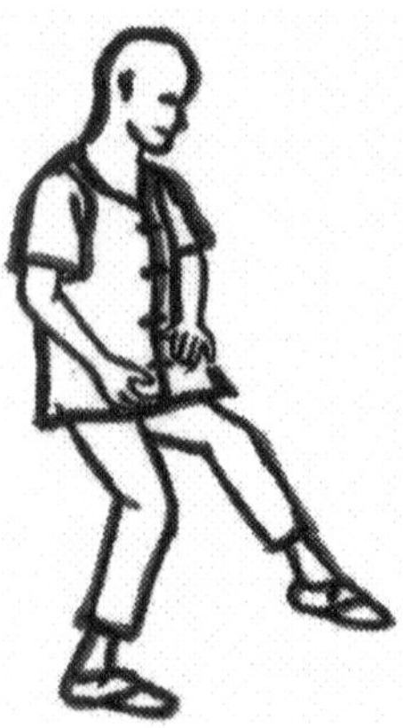

5. Raise both of your arms above your head and raise body and right leg forward at the same time, top and bottom together, on your left leg (1st time)
6. Keeping your right leg raised forward, lower both of your arms and body down, riding your left leg without letting your right toe touch down.
7. Again bring both of your arms and body and up on your left leg with right leg raised forward. (2nd time)
8. Lower your arms and body down on your left leg with your right leg still raised.
9. Again, raise both of your arms and body and up—top and bottom together—with right leg raised forward. (3rd time)
10. Lower your arms and body stopping arms at shoulder height and shoulder width and allowing your right foot (toe first) to touch down at the same time.
11. Sitting back on left leg, turn your waist 90 degrees to the left pivoting on right heel.
12. Shift your weight back onto the right leg, sit back lowering your arms and go down on your right leg.
13. Now raise both of your arms and your body up together on your right leg with your left leg raised forward. (1st time)
14. Keeping the left leg raised forward, lower your arms and body down, riding your right leg without allowing your left toe to touch down.
15. Bring both of your arms and body up on your right leg keeping your left leg raised forward. (2nd time)
16. Lower both of your arms and body down with your left leg raised forward—top and bottom together—on your right leg.

17. Raise body and both of your arms up on your right leg with your left leg raised forward. (3rd time)
18. Lower your arms and body allowing your arms to stop at shoulder height and shoulder width and your left foot (toe first) to touch down at the same time.
19. Turn your waist to the front pivoting left heel and evenly distribute your weight to the left adjusting right foot straight.
20. Sit and hold the ball.

Benefit:

This movement is an excellent exercise for balance—not only physical balance, but mind-body coordination for, in order to do this movement fluidly, you must keep your mind focused on your body center. This move, practiced anywhere during the work break or lunch hour, can act as a little island of rest and relaxation in a sea of turbulence.

The move's meditative aspects will energize you allowing you to easily cope with those little unpleasant distractions as they occur.

Movement 4a: Tiger Stepping-Right

1. From **Golden Phoenix Rising**, straighten your arms and fingers.
2. Shift your weight to the left.

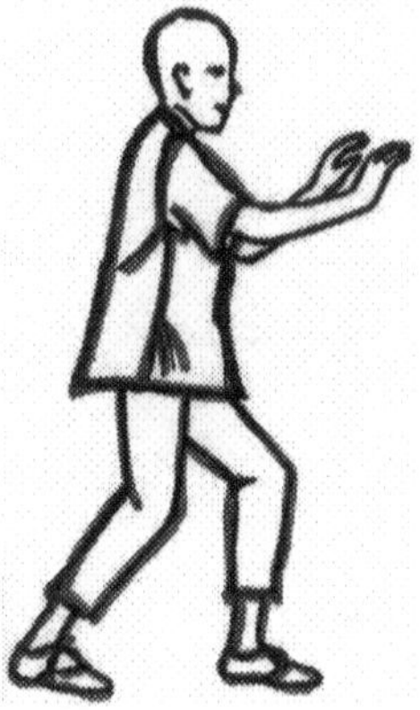

3. Bring your right toe in halfway.
4. Put the right foot down.
5. Raise your right toes and left heel.
6. Pivot 90 degrees to the right and line nose up with right toes.
7. Look down and go down.
8. Slowly come back up with same speed as going down.
9. Open your waist slightly to the right.
10. Sit back on left leg and step lightly with right leg.
11. Change weight to right leg and stand up—left foot follows naturally.
12. Bend your left knee, draw leg back and go down on right leg; raise your left leg forward and go up on right leg. (1st time)

13. Down (left leg back) and up (left leg forward) on right leg. (2nd time)
14. Down (left leg back) and up (left leg forward) on right leg. (3rd time)
15. On the 4th time down, place your left heel down with toes up.
16. Line your nose up with the toes of your left foot and look down as you go down.
17. With all of your weight on the back right leg, come back up at the same speed totally relaxed.
18. Open your waist slightly to the left; sit back on right leg and step lightly with left leg.
19. Change weight to the left leg and stand up—right foot follows naturally.
20. Bend your right knee, draw the leg back and go down on left leg; raise your right leg forward and go up on left leg. (1st time)
21. Down (right leg back) and up (right leg forward) on left leg. (2nd time)
22. Down (right leg back) and up (right leg forward) on left leg. (3rd time)
23. On 4th time down place the right heel down with toes up.
24. Line your nose up with toes of your right foot and look down as you go down.
25. With all of the weight on the back leg, come back up at the same speed relaxed.
26. When your body is straight, sit and turn your waist 180 degrees to the left, pivoting on your right foot.

Movement 4b: Tiger Stepping-Left

1. Change weight to the right leg—pick up the left toe and keep turning, pull left leg back and stand up.
2. Bend the left knee, draw the leg back and go down on right leg; raise your left leg forward and go up on right leg. (1st time)
3. Go down (left leg back) and stand up (left leg forward) on right leg. (2nd time)
4. Go down (left leg back) and stand up (left leg forward) on right leg. (3rd time)
5. On 4th time down place left heel down with toes up.

6. Line your nose up with the toes of your left foot and look down as you go down.

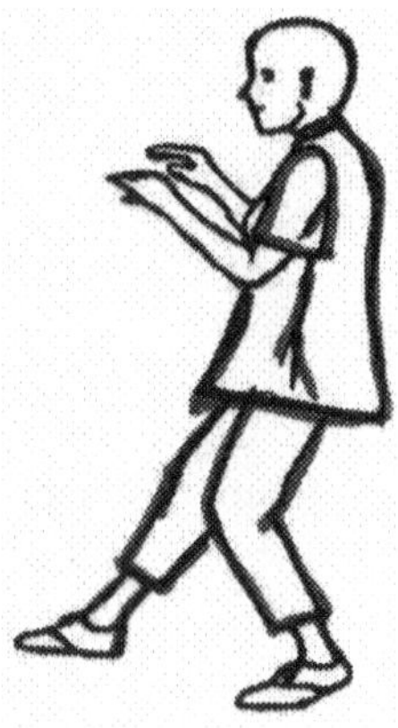

7. With all of your weight on the back leg; come back up, completely relaxed.
8. Turn the waist to the left a little; sit back on right leg and step lightly with left leg.
9. Change your weight to the left leg and stand up—right foot follows naturally.
10. Again, bend your right knee, draw the leg back and go down on left leg; raise your right leg forward and go up on left leg. (1st time)
11. Go down (right leg back) and up (right leg forward) on left leg. (2nd time)
12. Again, down (right leg back) and up (right leg back) on left leg. (3rd time)
13. On 4th time down, place right heel down with toes up.
14. Line nose up with toes of right foot and look down ad you go down
15. Come back up slowly and relaxed with all of your weight on your back leg.

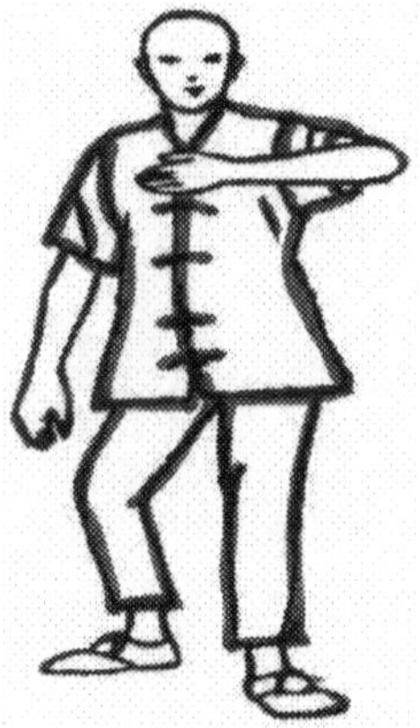

16. Open your waist slightly to the right; sit back on left leg and step lightly with right leg.
17. Change weight to the right leg and stand up—left foot follows naturally.
18. Again, bend your left knee, draw leg back and go down on right leg; raise your left leg forward and go up on right leg. (1st time)
19. Go down (left leg back) and up (left leg forward) on right leg. (2nd time)
20. Bend the right knee and go down (left leg back) and up (left leg forward). (3rd time)
21. On 4th time down, place left heel down with toes up.
22. Line nose up with toes of left foot and look down as you go down.
23. With all of the weight on the back leg and toes of front foot up, come back up slowly and relaxed.

24. From here, turn your waist back to the center pivoting on left heel and shift your weight to the left.
25. Pick up right toe and straighten right foot; place hands and fingers in front of the thighs.
26. Raise your arms to shoulder height and shoulder width and sit and hold the ball.

Benefit:

Next to lower back pain, sciatica brings more people to their knees than prayer and hampers normal activity from boardroom to bedroom. This tiger-stepping movement stretches the hamstring, ankle and instep while strengthening the muscles of the buttocks. All of this leads to more flexibility and suppleness than you've ever known before. You may find yourself eager to do things you haven't thought possible in years and notice enhanced sexual performance. Perhaps that is why they call it *Tiger Stepping.*

Movement 5: Embrace Tiger Return to Mountain

1. From here straighten your arms and fingers.
2. As your legs stand up and your arms straighten up above your head, turn palms out.

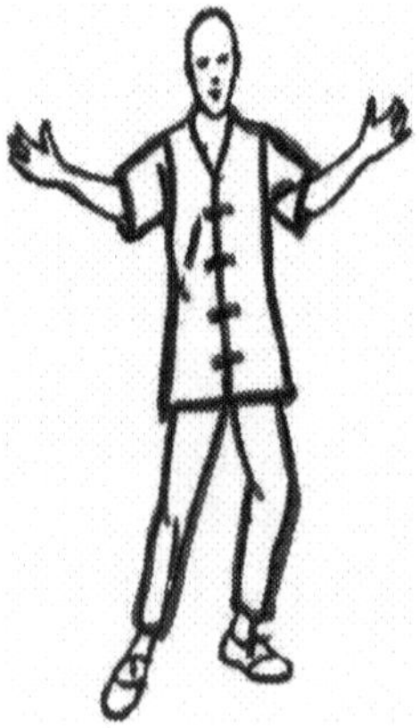

3. Continue your arms in a downward circle.
4. As your arms pass shoulder height, bend your wrists and knees at the same time.
5. Allow top and bottom to continue to go down together.
6. As your body stops, allow the inside of your wrists to brush both knees dropping your head.
7. Looking at your palms lay your right palm inside your left palm.
8. Turn your fingers away from the body and slowly stand up.
9. When your body is straight, turn the right palm up into a knife hand and slide hand through thumb and forefinger of left hand.
10. Turn both palms to face the earth.

11. Bring the right fingers to the left without touching and sit and hold the ball.

Repeat the entire sequence a second time:

1. From here, again, straighten the arms and fingers.
2. Legs stand up and arms go up above head at the same time.
3. Palms turn outward and arms continue in a downward circle.
4. As the wrists bend, also bend the knees at the same time.
5. Allow the top and bottom to go down together.
6. As your body stops, allow the inside of your wrists to brush both knees dropping your head.
7. Looking at your palms lay your right palm inside your left palm.
8. Turn your fingers away from the body and slowly stand up.

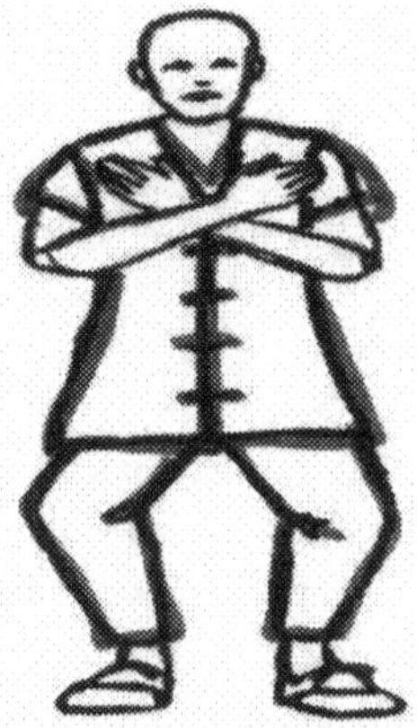

9. When your body is straight, turn the right palm up into a knife hand and slide hand through thumb and forefinger of left hand.
10. Turn both palms to face the earth.
11. Bring the right fingers to the left without touching and sit and hold the ball.

Now repeat the entire sequence a third and final time:

1. From here, again, straighten the arms and fingers.
2. Legs stand up and arms go up above the head at the same time.
3. Palms turn outward and arms continue in a downward circle.
4. When then wrists bend, bend the knees at the same time.
5. Allow the top and bottom to go down together.
6. As your body stops, allow the inside of your wrists to brush both knees dropping your head.
7. Looking at your palms lay your right palm inside your left palm.
8. Turn your fingers away from the body and slowly stand up.

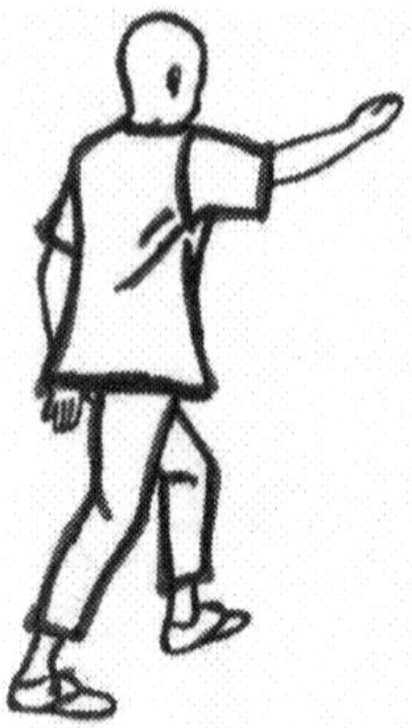

9. When your body is straight, turn the right palm up into a knife hand and slide hand through thumb and forefinger of left hand.
10. Turn both palms to face the earth.
11. Bring the right fingers to the left without touching and sit and hold the ball.

Benefit:

If conversation is an art, then graphic peer-group discussions on the difficulty of moving one's bowels can be called an exclusive western art form. Inadequate circulation of blood and energy to the lower intestines are the main causes of this problem. The simple exercise you are now watching, when combined with deep natural breathing, will allow you to be forever apathetic to all of those TV commercials dealing with the problems of irregularity and will enhance whole body circulation. Improper circulation obstructs all internal organs. Proper movement is derived only from proper balance and proper balance is created from the healthy flow of blood and breath.

Movement 6: Turning the Waist

1. From end of **Embrace Tiger Return to Mountain**, straighten your arms and fingers.
2. Shift your weight to the right.
3. Sink your body and step wide with your left toe and place left foot down.
4. Let your arms drop in front of the body.
5. From the waist, turn to the left and turn back past center to the right. (1st time)
6. With just the waist moving, turn to the left and back past center to the right. (2nd time)
7. Again, turn your waist to the left and back past center to the right. (3rd time)
8. Turn your waist back to center with arms in front of your body.

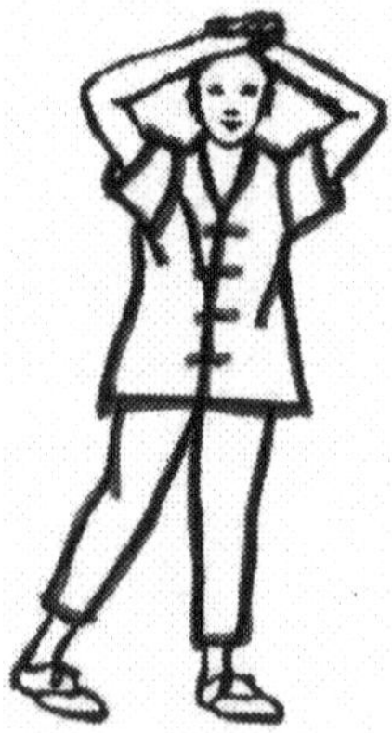

Benefit:

This move, which is expressly designed for massaging the kidneys by separating negative and positive (*Yin* and

Yang), has many added benefits for the weekend athlete. By distinguishing the difference between waist and hips, don't be surprised if your golf scores go down while the level of your tennis game comes up.

Movement 7: Collecting the energy

1. From **Turning the Waist**, change weight to the right leg.
2. Bring your left toe in 3 or 4 inches from right foot and lift your left leg and arms up and step like cat bringing arms down.
3. Change weight to your left leg.
4. Right leg only comes up and knee bends; step like a cat.
5. Change weight softly to right leg.
6. Both arms and left leg come up at the same time; and down together stepping like a cat.
7. Change weight to left leg.
8. Right leg comes up and knee bends; step like a cat.
9. Shift weight to the right leg.

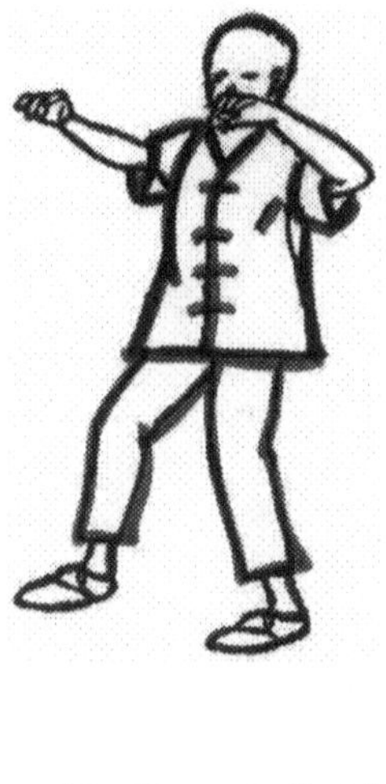

10. Both arms and left leg up same time; and down together stepping like a cat.
11. Change weight softly to left leg.
12. Right leg only comes up with knee bent and step like a cat.
13. Change weight to right softly.
14. Both arms and left leg with knee bent come up at same time.
15. Fingers face each other but do not touch.
16. Arms and leg come down together.
17. Place feet together and at the same time place hands at side.
18. Form is finished; slight bow.

Benefit:

This final movement gently gathers the energy and returns it to the *dan tian*, or body center and balances the brain. If the time spent with your arm in a blood pressure machine at the supermarket was spent instead on releasing the stress using this movement called *Collecting the Energy*, you would save a lot more than just those quarters.

He who distinguishes the true savor of his food can never be a glutton; he who does not cannot be otherwise.

–Henry David Thoreau

9

Tai Chi and Diet

Tell me what you eat, I'll tell you who you are.

–Anthelme Brillat-Savarin

The more you eat, the less flavor; the less you eat, the more flavor.

–Chinese Proverb

Pardon me, but I made an exception here since I found many appropriate quotes concerning foods. However, these three openers encapsulate much that I believe about why the foods we eat are so important. Over the past fifty years, our society has consistently moved away from growing wholesome vegetables and raising farm-fed animals. Today's processed foods are not the organic, healthy foods that our ancestors and grandparents ate. The chemicals and additives (preservatives, food colorings, etc.) added to processed foods have greatly weakened the benefits of most of the foods we consume. Even food that is grown in the earth has been contaminated by pesticides and environmental carelessness that is passed on to the feed provided for the animals. Although we have quite a selection of vitamins, minerals, and supplements in various other forms, our diet is still the most powerful determinant in our physical make-up. Food ought to provide us with all of the vitamins, minerals, proteins and carbohydrates necessary for proper nourishment. Often, correcting our diet can cure a dysfunction in our body while poor dietary habits can render other types of treatment ineffective. Because of that, obtaining a general knowledge of nutrition is essential to good health.

In his book, *Staying Healthy with the Seasons, 21st Century Edition*, Dr. Elson M. Haas has explored, in great detail, dietary habits leading to good health. He states, "Many of us live at a level that is not sick, but we're not really healthy either." He goes on to explain how the average American diet, being high in refined flour, sugar, fats and other ingredients, keeps the average American on the "not healthy" side of the wellness/illness continuum. According to him, appreciating the difference between "feeling healthy" and "not sick" is a matter of the choices we make. Certainly, healthful foods have always been an integral part of healthy living in Chinese medicine. Tai Chi is often a choice for those desiring to reduce stress levels in their daily living. Another factor to consider regarding our diet is that what we eat can actually increase our levels of stress; therefore, being aware of the right food to eat will dramatically improve our ability to cope during stressful times. Food is the body's fuel; how we digest, assimilate, and use the nutrients in our diets create the energy on which our body operates. Therefore, in relation to Tai Chi, food is one of the most important sources of life energy or *chi*. Good Tai Chi necessitates that our diets observe the optimum quantity and quality of *chi* taken into the body during the digestive process by eating the right mix of foods. We receive *chi* from each meal because each food has its own *yin* and *yang* energy content. Certain foods are rich in their supply of *chi* while other foods are nearly void of *chi*. Look at the difference between a plate of fresh fruits and vegetables and a plate of canned fruits and vegetables to see the difference in life energy content. We deplete food of its health-giving life energy by boiling, overcooking, canning, etc. Ultimately, the processing of food weakens the supply of *chi* available to the body. Most meat comes from animals injected with steroids or other hormones that serve to destroy its value. In fact, we are learning that processed foods, sprayed crops, and injected cattle and poultry may be more dangerous than we ever thought. Any chemical or additive in excess acts as a poison to the body. Even water treated with chemicals such as fluoride or chlorine may eventually harm those who drink it.

What other factors drain our body of *chi* and contribute to the overall reduced benefits of our diets? The air we breathe is part of our diet. Air polluted with exhaust fumes, industrial waste, or radiation is poisonous to all who inhale it. Drugs (alcohol, nicotine, caffeine, etc.) if used continuously or recklessly can also contaminate the body and will act as any other poison in our system. The two greatest incidences of disease today are cancer and heart disease. It is easy to see why after looking at what the average person consumes daily. Almost all packaged foods bought in supermarkets contain those additives and preservatives mentioned earlier as well as sugar and salt. The consumer must develop the habit of reading the ingredients on the label of each item and becoming familiar with the effects of these additives before deciding to make a purchase. I believe that, apart from genetics, cancer is the body's reaction to all the poisons that enter and irritate it.

Students often ask me about diet and what foods to avoid. Whether you should eat meat or be a vegetarian is an individual decision. Your personal needs, where you live, and your daily activity all contribute to what is right for you. Your upbringing and your culture also greatly influence your diet. I spend a great deal of time talking with African Americans about the diet of our culture and the things we can do to improve our health. The following list is a general compilation that I have collected over the years. It may be useful to anyone interested in preserving good health. At the close of this chapter, I will give details concerning my personal choices in diet and nutrition with any modifications I have made. My general list includes:

- ❖ Additives including preservatives, artificial colorings and flavorings, etc.: These build up in the body to form powerful toxins causing problematic disorders. (Special note to Tai Chi students: at your favorite Chinese restaurant, specify 'no M.S.G.' and limit your intake of tea or coffee.)
- ❖ Bleached or Polished Flour: This is flour stripped of its nutritional value and its life energy as well. Buy only whole grain breads and cakes with no preservatives added. Grains should constitute a large portion of one's diet.
- ❖ Polished Rice: Like processed flour, polished rice is nearly void of nutritional content. This is especially serious in underdeveloped countries where malnutrition is a problem. Eat brown rice.
- ❖ Refined Sugar (sucrose): Most sugar available today is refined sugar having no nutritional value. (I include brown sugar, artificial sweeteners or product containing them in this ban.) It contributes to vascular disorders, hypoglycemia, obesity, diabetes, and possibly cancer when consumed in large quantities. Replace needed sugar with honey, molasses, or real maple syrup
- ❖ Salt: Common table salt is 99% $NaCl$—a poison in large doses. Almost every food product has salt added to it. It is a major factor in high blood pressure, heart attacks, nervousness, and anxiety. Use only sea salt (or kelp) sparingly; sea salt contains only 1.5% $NaCl$ while nutrients make up the remaining contents.
- ❖ Fats: Margarine and the fats found in anything fried are among the worst of the 'bad' fats. When you see 'partially hydrogenated' on any food label,

avoid it. Refined vegetable oils are also on the 'bad' fats list because they oxidize easily. The use of high heat to process them removed all of the healthy nutrients like Vitamin E. (Extra virgin cold-pressed olive oil, however, is a 'good' fat and imparts a nice flavor but it cannot be heated as high as other oils. Canola oil is good to use on baking pans, waffle irons or other very hot utensils to keep food from sticking. Lowering both salt and fat intake helps to minimize heart disease.

- Caffeine: Coffee, tea, and colas contain caffeine. Caffeine is a stimulant. Is it any wonder that many children of the 'Cola-generation' are hyperactive and difficult to manage? Caffeine also destroys Vitamin B.
- Meats and poultry: Most meats and poultry contain steroids or other hormones considered very high contributors to cancer. Red meat contains 40% fat and takes an excessively long time to digest. This may irritate the digestive tract and may eventually result in cancer of the colon.

Begin by eating a balanced diet consisting of a variety of whole foods such as vegetables, fruits, milk, eggs, grains, legumes, nuts and seeds. If vitamins and other supplements are a part of your regimen, make sure they are those naturally extracted from foods and not those synthesized from chemicals. Choose 'good' fats. Good fats are the naturally occurring, traditional fats that have not been damaged by high heat, refining, processing or other fabricated tampering such as 'partial hydrogenation'. The best of these kinds of fats are found in fish, nuts, avocados, seeds and, unbelievably, fresh creamery butter. Certain essential fats such as omega-3s (found in oily fish) and the occasional omega-6 (found in evening primrose oil) treat everything from bipolar depression to skin problems. Some can even benefit us in weight-loss programs. If meat is not eliminated, then limit the amount consumed on a weekly basis; choose fish and poultry more often. Another simple yet often overlooked habit to maintain is that of chewing foods well. This seemingly unimportant act aids in digestion and is reputed to heighten the *chi* output in foods as well. The habit of overeating not only contributes to obesity but also diminishes the *chi* in the body. Therefore, stuffing the stomach at meals should not be the goal. Perhaps two meals a day is actually healthier than three; some diets recommend six small meals per day. A tidbit of advice I recall from one of my teachers is to fill 1/3 of the stomach with food and 1/3 with liquid while the remaining 1/3 should remain empty.

At any rate, the more conscious we become of our food consumption, the less we will contaminate ourselves with poisons and the more we will turn to a healthy diet as a rich source of the health-giving *chi*. Dr. Haas' common sense observations along with our discussion thus far may be summarized as follows:

- Nature provides us with foods that keep our bodies in balance with the climate
- We usually eat differently during winter than we eat during the summer
- Using diet to heat and cool the body is a good balancing tool for good health. Avoid extremely hot or cold/frozen foods or drinks since the stomach has to work harder to cool or warm its contents to the proper temperature
- Our bodies need extra food when we do physical work or exercise but during inactive times our food intake need to be less or else we will gain weight
- Eat moderately because eating too much is stressful on the body (even the good foods)
- East simply by avoiding mixing too many different foods at one meal; excessive and undigested foods lead to blockages, which stress the digestive system
- Chew food completely allowing our saliva to prepare the food for digestion (swallow when texture is creamy)
- Abstain from all harmful substances: alcohol, tobacco, coffee, tea (except herbal teas), drugs, soft drinks, etc.
- Eat early since eating close to sleep can lead to restlessness due to fermentation of undigested food; the stomach needs about four hours for proper digestion (Eating two meals a day, choose close to 8 a.m. and between 2p.m. and 3 p.m. allowing ample time between meals for the stomach to rest; Eating three meals a day, aim for 6:30 a.m., noon, and 5:30 p.m.)
- Live by the clock, especially during the first month of change, keeping to a schedule as much as possible: meals, bedtime, waking, study, work, prayers/meditation, physical hygiene, etc.
- Drink plenty of water

We can all follow Dr. Haas' recommendation to keep our nutrition light, wholesome, natural and seasonal. I believe, as he does, that seasonal eating promotes the health of not only our bodies but also that of the earth. As he points out, "staying healthy involves shifting taste buds and habits." A well-balanced diet generates quality *chi* increasing our vitality and establishing good health. I will close this chapter by making a few comments on my personal choices and outlining a sample menu for a day.

I have made a decision to avoid all refined foods, attempt to select the foods adequate for the intake of vitamins, minerals, and other nutrients, and choose those nutrients that will help maintain balanced weight while fighting the excesses of cholesterol and other unwanted materials that cause degeneration of the tissues. Some of the points of my personal choices and modifications are:

- Eat no flesh food or canned "fake" meat
- Use no dairy products including eggs, eggs products, butter, milk, hard and soft cheeses, cottage cheese, cream cheese, whey, etc.
- Read labels and buy nothing with chemicals listed as ingredients
- Use no vinegar or products containing it (ketchup, pickles, mayonnaise, salad dressings, etc.)
- Use no spices [allspice, cinnamon, clover, ginger, mustard seed, nutmeg, etc.], which are parts of trees or plants grown in topical regions (Herbs are fine as long as they are parts of plants that grow in temperate regions [e.g. basil, bay leaf, coriander, cilantro, cumin, dill, fennel, marjoram, mint, paprika, parsley, rosemary, saffron, sage, savory, tarragon, thyme, etc.])
- Use no irritating peppers (black, white, hot [jalapeños, chili, etc.], pepper sauces, etc.—bell, pimento, cherry, banana and other "not hot" peppers are permitted along with cayenne pepper)
- Use no baking soda or baking powder
- Eat only bread/crackers leavened with yeast or hydrogen peroxide or eat unleavened bread/crackers
- Eat no fried foods
- Eat nothing between meals (including chewing gum or "tasting" while preparing meals) since any food causes the mouth to produce saliva to aid the stomach in the digestive process-the stomach needs time to rest
- Drink no water with meals and plenty between meals
- Eat fruits, vegetables, nuts and seeds, legumes, and grains in as fresh a state as possible (frozen is next best; packed or canned in glass with fruit juice or water is also acceptable; dried is fine as well)
- Avoid irradiated produce

- Avoid cooking in aluminum (use stainless steel, corning ware or glass pots and pans)
- Avoid use of the microwave and pressure cooker (use the stove or oven as much as possible and do not overcook)
- Attempt to maintain an 80%/20% alkaline (acid binding elements)/acid (acid forming elements) ratio in my diet [Most fruits and vegetables are acid binding while most starches and proteins are acid forming; body organs and glands depend on secretions that are alkaline for optimal health]
- Do not mix fruits and vegetables at one meal

I often limit my intake to two meals per day but I will close with sample menus for three meals per day along with a few recipes. The best daily regimen for me to follow is to have two fruits (a citrus plus another—especially apples—preferably at breakfast), six vegetables (a yellow such carrots, a green, a legume, and a raw salad at both lunch and supper), and a protein and a starch (these may include two types of whole grains along with tubers and nuts)—one each at the lunch and evening meal. When following such a diet plan, I can receive all of my nutritional needs from the daily servings of these foods.

Breakfast is the important meal of the day as it "breaks the fast" from the previous hours of digestive inactivity. The body needs fuel to run for the day. The mid-day meal is also strategic in that it stokes the energy level begun at breakfast to maintain endurance throughout the remainder of the day. Vegetables and grains eaten at this meal create variety. The last meal of the day should be the lightest. We should leave a space of four to five hours prior to bedtime in order for the digestive process to complete. Doing this helps to eliminate certain gastric problems caused by allowing undigested food to remain in our stomachs throughout the night.

Sample Basic Menu for Good Chi

I. Breakfast

- Cooked grain (millet, brown rice, barley, rolled oats, buckwheat, etc.)
- Fresh fruits
- 8–10 Almonds
  or
  1 tablespoon sunflower seeds, pumpkin seeds, or sesame seeds
- Grain or Nut Milk*

Grain or Nut Milk

1 cup of cooked grains (e.g. millet or brown rice) **OR**
1 cup of raw nuts or seeds
2–3 cups of water (the amount determines the thickness)
Blend in blender until liquefied

II. Mid-day

- Cooked grain (brown rice, corn, millet) **OR**
  Red Potato (baked or boiled)
- Whole grain pasta
- Steamed green vegetable or cooked, fresh peas or beans
- Raw salad (leaf lettuce or romaine, carrots, celery, radishes, bell peppers, sprouts, etc.) with Lemon juice/honey dressing (omit honey if diabetic or low blood sugar)

Sunflower Seed Dressing

1 and 2/3 cups water
1 tsp. salt (optional)
½ tsp. onion powder
1 cup sunflower seeds
1/3 cup fresh lemon juice
Blend in blender until very creamy

III. Evening

- Vegetable soup with whole grain bread **OR**
  Fruit salad and bread **OR**
  Raw salad (same as mid-day except add salmon) and bread
- Big Mama's Sweet Potato Pie?—**NOT!** ☺

Hands Holding Taiji shakes the whole world,
A chest containing ultimate skill defeats a gathering of heroes.

– Written for Yang Lu Chan by Ong Tong He, scholar

10

Tai Chi FAQs

1. How early would you allow a child to begin Tai Chi?

   Because Tai Chi requires a certain level of coordination and concentration, I do not think it is appropriate for children. They usually need something faster, like karate, to help their bones and muscles develop and to keep their attention. Originally, those who studied Tai Chi were already students of other martial arts and Tai Chi advanced their level of skill. There may be exceptions but generally, I would not accept students for Tai Chi who are under eighteen.

2. Is Tai Chi by itself enough exercise?

   I often tell my students that Tai Chi is an initiation into exercise and better health. Tai Chi is neither an aerobic nor a muscle strength/endurance type of exercise. The stance used while performing the Tai Chi form does have an impact on the overall workout received. Although Tai Chi can be performed in a low, medium or high stance (with the low stance providing the highest workout intensity), it is generally performed in a medium to high stance while the low stance is reserved for Tai Chi adepts. The intensity of Tai Chi is often compared that of a low to moderate intensity aerobic exercise akin to brisk walking, and yet the cardiovascular results appear to be indicative of activities with higher training intensities. I would suggest that you first consider your specific goals from an exercise program. From this comparison, you should be able to gauge how Tai Chi would fit into your desired health regimen. However, while an hour of Tai Chi may bring the body into an aerobic state, typical practice is not in the aerobic range. As one Tai Chi practitioner and instructor put it, "It's not aerobic, but it loosens you up. It also complements other activities and sports."

3. Some of the movements appear to be painful. Are they?

   Let me repeat: Tai Chi is not practiced under the "no pain—no gain" mantra!! The defining characteristic of Tai Chi is its *gentleness*. You may have observed Tai Chi being performed in a low stance, which may look quite painful but rest assured that those practitioners are not novices and have both studied and practiced the art for a long time. A beginner would not be expected to assume those postures; your muscles will stretch and yield—without force—as you grow in the art. In addition, in many cases the instructor will modify exercises to prevent injury to those suffering from certain medical conditions. As part of a regular Tai Chi class, you will always begin with preliminary exercises to include breathing and stretching to create greater joint flexibility and stability thereby limiting the possibility of pain and injury. When practicing alone it is important to listen to your body and continue to practice proper posture along with those stretching and breathing exercises each time you practice.

4. How do I decide what style is for me?

   My first suggestion would be to find out what is available in your area. Do not decide by merely reading descriptions. Visit several schools, if possible. Talk to the instructors. Take the introductory session. Remember that all Tai Chi emerged from one source, so I would not be too concerned about which style to pursue unless a physical condition made the primary moves of a particular style restrictive. There are many different versions of Tai Chi but if they hold to the basic concepts mentioned elsewhere in this book, they are all valid.

5. How can I find Tai Chi classes?

   Tai Chi is now a part of many different environments: community extension classes, sports clubs and gyms, churches, and rehabilitation facilities. Although this may serve your purposes, do not expect the same rigor and discipline as that found in a Tai Chi school. You should find schools listed among the other martial arts or karate schools in your area. Even if no Tai Chi schools exist, call or visit the other martial arts schools and talk to the staff. They may be able to point you in the right direction.

6. What do I need in order to begin?

   Tai Chi requires no special clothing, equipment or practice space. One key thing that helps is perseverance. Beginning to learn the various movements may seem to go slowly and appear to be unproductive, but the results of being constant and building gradually will pay off. It is also important to practice mindfulness—being 100% present and focused on whatever the task may be. Mindfulness training, a meditation practice commonly found in Buddhism, is the technique of bringing awareness to the here and now. Apply this awareness to the sensations in your body instead of letting the awareness slip away into thoughts of the future or other issues. The assumption is that when you act with full awareness, your habits are more likely to achieve what you intend, and you will feel more fulfilled. Semiconsciously practicing Tai Chi without really focusing attention on the present moment or directing your attention toward things other than your practice time will not allow you to achieve your ultimate mastery. Unmindful practice may also result in failure to experience fully the sensory and healing benefits of Tai Chi. In order to break the habit of unmindful moving, take the moments of preparation, when you assume the initial stance, to appreciate fully its meaning and value before you begin the Tai Chi form. As you begin the first movement, try to give it your full attention. Savor each movement and enjoy the entire set of movements each time you practice.

7. Why do I need an instructor?

   A good instructor has the ability to learn, assimilate new knowledge, and then pass it on in such a way that others can understand. A good instructor wants his students to be more, not less, skillful than himself, so he will give anything they can learn with nothing held back. It is possible to watch videos and read books to enhance practice time, but learning with an instructor is the surest way of beginning the requisite skills correctly. Learning proper stances, correct body alignment and whole body coordination is difficult via reading books or watching videos and may lead to improper basics. This only helps perpetuate a lower quality of Tai Chi—perfect practice makes perfect quality. In reality, only constant, diligent practice and dedication will allow a student to learn, understand, and progress. The regular drilling of the positions received from a good instructor serves to make it easier to remember and connect those movements into a coordinated, fluid, whole-body form. A good instructor maintains a healthy environment for learning and receiving instant feedback.

8. How can I recognize a good instructor?

   The content as well as the quality of instruction in Tai Chi varies widely, so the best idea is to determine what your own objectives are before you begin looking for a school to help you fulfill them. Read good Tai Chi books. You can ask for a referral from other students or teachers. It is important to figure out why you are taking the class and make sure the class is suitable for your needs. Does a reputable master or organization certify the teacher or did they just study with someone for a while and then go off to teach? Is the teacher reputable? What is their lineage? Does the teacher have a bad temper? As a beginner, you will have very little to go on to find a good instructor. Sometimes great masters make terrible teachers, while some lower ranked teachers are better able to transfer the knowledge they have. Sometimes students benefit little from the master because they allow their advanced students to do all the teaching. So finding a good teacher may be as much up to chance as to research. One way to judge a teacher is by the students. If the students are of good technical quality and seem reasonably proficient, the instructor is most likely competent. Avoid teachers who do not allow visitors. In learning a Chinese art, the natural inclination is to look for a Chinese instructor. Let go of that expectation; it has drawbacks. One problem is that many Chinese instructors may not communicate very well in English. Another is that being Chinese does not automatically make the instructor excellent just as being non-Chinese does not automatically make the instructor or school mediocre!

9. How often should I practice?

   In order to gain maximum benefit from Tai Chi, practice must be daily. At first, simply learning the postures and remembering them from day to day will seem to be a lot to do. Once you can put it all together, then practicing daily is the only way to continue to develop the skills. Actually, practicing several times a day is not unheard of since it takes a relatively short amount of time to do the form. Health appraisals of some Tai Chi practitioners who have practiced Tai Chi for seven years or more show that most of them practice Tai Chi as their only form of regular exercise. They perform it slowly at a low to medium stance with a moderate to high level of intensity with for one hour and an average frequency of seven times a week.

10. What can I expect to pay?

    The Tai Chi form is usually broken into parts and the individual school sets the fees accordingly. The cost for Tai Chi classes is comparable to any of the other martial arts classes. The formal class session usually lasts for one hour and is held once or twice a week at a specified time. There is also private instruction available with prices set by the instructor.

11. How long should I take instruction?

    Formal instruction may last for years. People study Tai Chi for various reasons, including for its health benefits and mystical/spiritual benefits. Each goal has its own training emphasis. For example, if you were interested in the health benefit, to reap the benefits of this art you would need to practice 30 to 60 minutes, three to six days per week. Obviously, this includes both the time spent with an instructor and the time spent on your own. The health benefits start at about 10 minutes, but if you practice 20 to 60 minutes per session you will get maximum benefits. Up to a point, there is a direct relationship between how long a student takes lessons and his skill level. Previous training and innate talent are also major factors. Some experts claim that the time spent in the art does not necessarily correlate to skill. This is because there are many people who practice Tai Chi all their lives and do not show any *kung-fu* skill. Nevertheless, they still will get the health benefits from doing the exercise. Learning Tai Chi is a systematic process. There is a correlation between skill and the amount of time spent studying **correctly** in a structured class. To progress on the martial side of the art, the student must do certain art specific partner training methods. Those not interested in that can perform the art and gain the health and meditation benefits. There are many ways to practice. It is a life-long, recursive developmental process.

12. What is the ranking system in Tai Chi?

    If you are thinking of other forms of the martial arts that incorporate belts and degrees in moving from one competency level to another, then Tai Chi does not fit into that. Tai Chi is about self-mastery and does not use belts and degrees. Individual teachers, however, will use a system of colors to rank *their* students as they move through various forms and demonstrate skills and knowledge. Students wear these colors as sashes around the waist or as tops during practice time to represent the increasing commitment and observable improvement in the practice of Tai Chi. Traditionally, the Chinese arts rank students in a familial type of rank such as older brother, younger brother, and so forth. Although some traditional schools reward competence by giving a diploma, usually a student receives a certificate or formal permission to teach others once he/she reaches a certain level of competence.

13. How can I compete in Tai Chi?

    Because Tai Chi does not use belts or degrees, at competitions students compete in standardized style, weapons forms, and push hands with an opponent. The competitions usually take place in three separate areas. The area for push hands is normally an elevated platform. Contestants score on the flow of their movements, balance, flexibility, coordination, elegance, techniques (eye, hand, foot, etc.) used, internal energy, and power. The person with the highest score wins. In push hands, the contestant who does not fall from the platform wins. Your instructor will be able to give you more information as the time for each competition draws near.

14. What is the significance of touching the tongue to the roof of the mouth as we practice the Tai Chi form?

    As we talked earlier about how *chi* circulates through the body, we mentioned that it travels along meridians or channels through the body. The idea is to form a closed circuit within the body as it generates and moves *chi*. According to Mantak Chia in *Iron Shirt Chi Kung I* (1986), pp. 68-70, "the ancient Taoist Masters discovered that there were many channels to which energy can flow." However, two of them carry especially strong currents. One of these channels is the *functional* channel. It begins at the perineum, the point located at the base of the trunk midway between the testicles/vagina and the anus, goes up the front of the body past the sex organs, stomach, heart, throat and stops at the pit of the tongue. The second, called the *governor* channel, also starts at the perineum but works upward along the back of the body past the tailbone, sacral pump, through the spine, into the brain and the cranial pump, finally flowing back down to the roof of the mouth. The tongue is similar to a switch controlling these two currents and when it is touched to the roof of the mouth (just behind the teeth), the energy can flow in a pattern up the spine and back down the front completing the circuit. This created loop of energy, or microcosmic orbit, flows past all of the major organs and nervous system of the body giving growing, healing and functioning energy to each of the cells. The governor channel guides the *chi* up the back and then the functional channel brings it down the front of the body completing the circuit where it once again becomes the governor channel, and so on. Mantak Chia has named this path the *microcosmic orbit.*

15. I think I can see how some of the movements in *The Seven Golden Movements* correlate to particular movements in the Yang form, but can you give me the health benefits of a few of the movements we know from the Yang form?

    You already know how the *chi* moves through the body, therefore, the colon and elimination organs are involved first, followed by the kidneys, liver, lungs, and on upward culminating with the mind. Tai Chi also helps to circulate the lymph throughout the body via movements focused on lymph gland locations in the neck, armpits, elbows, knees and groin. Additionally, the movements of Tai Chi foster flexibility in the movement of the body. Although you may find information elsewhere that more fully discusses the benefits of the various movements, following is a list of some of the basic movements from the Yang long form and the health benefits for the related body organs and members as taught to me by my teachers:

    Beginning (Grasp Sparrow's Tail/Rollback/Press/Withdraw/Push)—this group aids the elimination organs of the digestive system (colon, large intestine, etc.)
    Single Whip—helps the lungs; opens all joints in the body; aids digestive system
    Lift Hands/Play Guitar—beneficial for the liver
    White Crane Spreads Wings—aids the lymph glands, vertebrae and central nervous system
    Brush Knee and Twist Step—helps the lower digestive tract, heart and stomach
    Step Forward, Deflect Downward, Parry, and Punch—this group helps the glands, strengthens the legs, and aids in the flexibility of the lower back
    Apparent Closure and Push; Carry Tiger and Return to Mountain—assist gastric-intestinal functions and rejuvenates the organs
    Step Back and Repulse Monkey—beneficial to the gall bladder and spinal cord
    Diagonal Flying—aids the lungs and small intestine
    Pick Up Needle at Sea Bottom—also beneficial for the liver as well as the spine and sexual organs
    Fan Through the Back—beneficial to small intestine

Wave Hands Like Clouds—aids the stomach area including the spleen and pancreas
High Pat on Horse—helps the spleen
Separate Right and Left Foot—balances excessive *yang* energy in the body
Turn and Kick with Left Heel—beneficial for the kidneys and stomach
Right Heel Kick—helps the kidneys and stomach
Hit Tiger Left and Right—helps the back
Parting Wild Horse's Mane—assists the lungs and spleen
Fair Lady Works at Shuttles—invigorates the chest area
Snake Creeps Down—beneficial to the kidneys and aids in general body flexibility
Golden Cock Stands on One Leg—helps improve stomach disorders
Step Up to Seven Stars—aids blood circulation
Turn and Sweep Lotus—Activates *yang* energy and balances *yin* dullness
Bend Bow and Shoot Tiger—aids the lungs

16. What level of physical fitness do I need before beginning Tai Chi?

    First, be sure that you have your doctor's permission to begin. After that, there are no restrictions. In fact, many of the Tai Chi movements have even been adapted to wheelchair users with accompanying individual attention. You should also let your instructor know of any disability that may restrict certain movements.

    I also stress avoiding heavy meals before Tai Chi practice to keep the body fit as well as avoiding eating or drinking immediately after practice. If you have not eaten, I recommend eating a light meal since you should also avoid practicing on an empty stomach. You should be fit enough to keep moving for a few minutes after practice to allow the pulse to return to normal. If you find that you are tired after practice, consult your doctor.

    Finally, make sure that you drink enough water during the day and get enough rest at night. As we practice Tai Chi, our bodies purge toxins and it is important to irrigate the body with enough water daily. (I recommend one and a half to two liters each day.) Sleep rejuvenates our bodies, helps our concentration, and aids in the health of our immune system.

17. What would you recommend as the best time to practice Tai Chi?

    Since the time to complete Tai Chi practice is not long, you can find time at almost any hour of the day during your spare time. However, I teach my students as my teachers taught me—the best times are in the morning just after sunrise and in the evening just before sunset. I oftentimes simplify this to be half an hour after rising or one hour before retiring. Along with the best times to practice and the comments on diet and rest already mentioned, I offer the following for your consideration as well in order to preserve *chi* and not block it:

- Do not practice Tai Chi during electrical storm activity. As we root, we become natural lightening rods.
- Do not practice in the direct mid-day sunlight. If practice does occur at mid-day, be sure to be in the shade out of the direct sunlight.
- Do not practice with barefoot on a cold hard surface. A cold surface will draw *chi* from the body.
- Do not drink alcohol (or take other drugs) before practice.

In this last chapter, I tried to address some of the questions and concerns that may make it easier for you to decide to learn more about Tai Chi. I want to close with a final quotation, an excerpt from the teachings of Master Lao Tzu as recorded in the Hua Hu Ching, chapter 38:

Why scurry about looking for the truth?
It vibrates in every thing and every not-thing, right off the tip of your nose.
Can you be still and see it in the mountain? the pine tree? yourself?
Don't imagine that you'll discover it by accumulating more knowledge.
Knowledge creates doubt, and doubt makes you ravenous for more knowledge.
You can't get full eating this way.
The wise person dines on something more subtle:
He eats the understanding that the named was born from the unnamed, that all being flows from non-being, that the describable world emanates from an indescribable source.
He finds this subtle truth inside his own self, and becomes completely content.
So who can be still and watch the chess game of the world?
The foolish are always making impulsive moves, but the wise know that victory and defeat are decided by something more subtle.
They see that something perfect exists before any move is made.
This subtle perfection deteriorates when artificial actions are taken, so be content not to disturb the peace.
Remain quiet.
Discover the harmony in your own being. Embrace it.

If you can do this, you will gain everything, and the world will become healthy again.
If you can't, you will be lost in the shadows forever.

I continue to search for my next teacher. Peace and blessings. Sankofa.

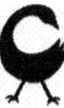

Bibliography

Books

Albin, Melanie. *Total Wellness: How to Live a Peaceful and Harmonious Life.* Melanie Albin. 2002

Ashby, Muata. *Egyptian Yoga: The Philosophy of Enlightenment (2nd Edition).* Cruzian Mystic Books. 1997.

Chandler, Wayne B. *Ancient Future.* Black Classic Press. 1999.

Chia, Mantak et al. *Awaken the Healing Light of the Tao.* Charles E. Tuttle Co. 1993.

Chu, Vincent. *Beginner's Tai Chi Chuan.* Unique Publications. 2000.

Chuen, Lam Kam. *Step-by-Step Tai Chi.* Fireside Books. 1994.

Dang, Tri Thong. *Beginning Tai Chi.* Charles E Tuttle Co. 1994.

Douglas, Bill. *The Complete Idiot's Guide to T'ai Chi & QiGong (2nd Edition).* Alpha Books. 2002.

Haas, Elson M. *Staying Healthy With the Season, 21st Century Edition.* Celestial Arts. 2003.

Hay, Louise L. *Heal Your Body: The Mental Causes for Physical Illness and The Metaphysical Way to Overcome Them.* Hay House. 1988.

Jahnke, Roger. *The Healing Promise of Qi: Creating Extraordinary Wellness through Qigong and Tai Chi.* McGraw Hill/Contemporary Books. 2002.

Lacouperie, T de. *The Languages of China before the Chinese.* London: David Nutt. 1887. (Reprint, 1970.)

Liao, Waysun. *Tai Chi Classics.* Shambhala Classics. 2000.

Little and Wong. *The Ultimate Guide to Tai Chi: The Best of Inside Kung-Fu.* Contemporary Books. 2000.

Lynch and Chungliang. *Thinking Body, Dancing Mind.* Bantam Doubleday Dell. 1994.

Maasi and Salim. *Kupigana Ngumi: Root Symbols of the Ntchru and Ancient Kemet, Vol. I.* Pan-Afrakan Kupigana Ngumi Press/Black Gold Press. 1992.

Means, Rev. Sterling M. *Ethiopia and the Missing Link in African History.* Lushena Books. 2001.

Rashidi and Sertima. *African Presence in Early Asia (10th Anniversary Edition).* Transaction Publishers. 2002.

Reed, Daniel P. *The Tao of Health, Sex and Longevity: A Modern Practical Guide to the Ancient Way.* Fireside Books/Simon & Schuster. 1987.

Rodgers, J. A. *100 Amazing Facts About the Negro with Complete Proof: A Short Cut to the World History of the Negro.* Helga Rodgers. 1995.

Articles

Allan, S. *Sons of Suns: Myth and Totemism in Early China.* Bulletin of the School of Oriental and African Studies (BSOAS) XLIV,(1981) pages 290-326.

McKay, Ken. *The Effects of Holistic Treatment Methods on Stress Related Illness.* University of Illinois. 2002.

Winters, Clyde Ahmad. *Blacks in Ancient China, Part 1: The Founders of Xia and Shang.* Journal of Black Studies 1, No. 2 (1983c).

Winters, Clyde Ahmad. *The Indus Valley Writing and related Scripts of the 3rd Millennium BC.* India Past and Present 2, no1 (1985b), pages 13-19.

Journals and Newsletters

The Annals of Behavioral Medicine, 2001; Vol. 23:139-146

The CIGNA newsletter, *Wellbeing*, winter, 1998

The Harvard Woman's Health Watch, Dec 2000, article, *"Tai Chi: Meditative movement for Health"*

The University of California, Berkeley, *Wellness Letter*, 1998

Other Resources

Candida, Gluten, and Diet, http://www.CandidaPage.com/weisscgd.shtml
Abstracts of Tai Chi Studies: 1976–1996,

http://www.taichiacademy.com/healthabstract7696.htm

About the Author

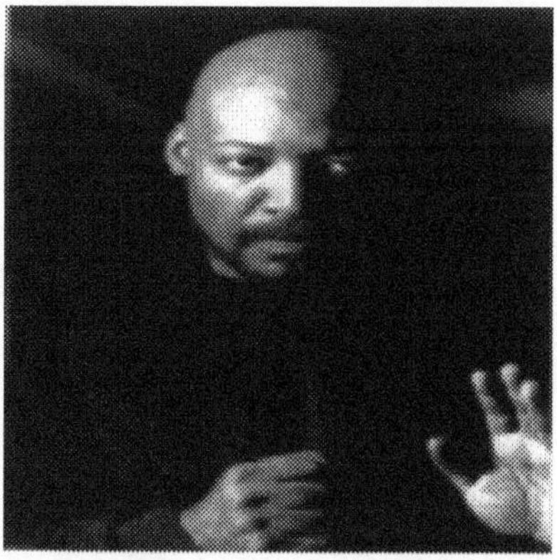

Mfundishi Obuabasa Serikali holds memberships in several national and international Tai Chi organizations including the International Yang Style Tai Chi Chuan Association and the American Yangjia Michuan Tajiquan Association. He is currently certified as a Tai Chi instructor by the National Wellness Institute through the Metro Louisville (KY) Health Department. The martial sciences have been a central part of the life of Mfundishi Obuabasa Serikali for over 40 years. In addition to Tai Chi Chuan, Mfundishi Serikali has taught meditation, yoga, and karate. As a lifelong resident of Louisville, Kentucky, he has devoted his life to extend the discipline of the arts to all people. After 27 years of service, he retired from the City of Louisville in 1999 where he also rendered service as a gang coordinator for the City of Louisville. Having received certification in Stress Management, he has worked with individuals and groups from all lifestyles to bring about increased awareness of the effects of stress through his Tai Chi classes. Coupled with his desire to motivate others to improve their health through diet and exercise, Mfundishi Serikali lectures throughout Louisville on the topics of wellness, stress management, and spirituality as well. Along with regular classes and workshops on Tai Chi, he has firmly committed himself to helping others, especially those who previously led a sedentary lifestyle, realize their maximum potential and live their lives in a more healthy way. To that end, his Tai Chi program has been included in phase I of the Mayor's Healthy Hometown Movement. This is a community-wide effort to create a new culture in Louisville where physical activity and optimal nutrition are the norm.

978-0-595-39857-7
0-595-39857-X

www.ingramcontent.com/pod-product-compliance
Lightning Source LLC
Chambersburg PA
CBHW051422280526
45785CB00003B/1125
* 9 7 8 0 5 9 5 3 9 8 5 7 7 *